Haematology at a Glance

Haematology at a Glance

ATUL B. MEHTA
MA MD FRCP FRCPath
Royal Free and University College School of Medicine
Royal Free Hospital
London
NW3 2QG

A. VICTOR HOFFBRAND
MA DM FRCP FRCPath FRCP (Edin) DSc
Royal Free and University College School of Medicine
Royal Free Hospital
London
NW3 2QG

b
Blackwell
Science

© 2000 by
Blackwell Science Ltd
Editorial Offices:
Osney Mead, Oxford OX2 0EL
25 John Street, London WC1N 2BS
23 Ainslie Place, Edinburgh EH3 6AJ
350 Main Street, Malden
   MA 02148-5018, USA
54 University Street, Carlton
   Victoria 3053, Australia
10, rue Casimir Delavigne
   75006 Paris, France

Other Editorial Offices:
Blackwell Wissenschafts-Verlag GmbH
Kurfürstendamm 57
10707 Berlin, Germany

Blackwell Science KK
MG Kodenmacho Building
7–10 Kodenmacho Nihombashi
Chuo-ku, Tokyo 104, Japan

Iowa State University Press
A Blackwell Science Company
2121 S. State Avenue
Ames, Iowa 50014-8300, USA

First published 2000
Reprinted 2000, 2001

Set by Excel Typesetters, Hong Kong
Printed and bound in Italy by G. Canale &
C. SpA, Turin

The Blackwell Science logo is a
trade mark of Blackwell Science Ltd,
registered at the United Kingdom
Trade Marks Registry

A catalogue record for this title
is available from the British Library

ISBN 0-632-04793-3

Library of Congress
Cataloging-in-publication Data

Mehta, A.B.
   Haematology at a glance/Atul Mehta, Victor
Hoffbrand.
      p   cm.
   Includes bibliographical references and index.
   ISBN 0-632-04793-3
   1. Hematology—Handbooks, manuals,
etc.   2. Blood—Diseases—Handbooks,
manuals, etc.   I. Title.   II. Mehta, Atul.
   [DNLM: 1. Hematologic Diseases.
   2. Blood Cells—cytology. WH 120 H698h
2000]   RB145 .H57 2000
   616.1'521—dc21

                              99-040674

DISTRIBUTORS

   Marston Book Services Ltd
   PO Box 269
   Abingdon, Oxon OX14 4YN
   (Orders: Tel: 01235 465500
             Fax: 01235 465555)

The Americas
   Blackwell Publishing
   c/o AIDC
   PO Box 20
   50 Winter Sport Lane
   Williston, VT 05495-0020
   (Orders: Tel: 800 216 2522
             Fax: 802 864 7626)

Australia
   Blackwell Science Pty Ltd
   54 University Street
   Carlton, Victoria 3053
   (Orders: Tel: 3 9347 0300
             Fax: 3 9347 5001)

For further information on
Blackwell Science, visit our website:
www.blackwell-science.com

Contents

Preface

With the ever-increasing complexity of the medical under-graduate curriculum, we feel that there is a need for a concise introduction to clinical and laboratory haematology for medical students. The *At a Glance* format has allowed us to divide the subject into easily digestible slices or bytes of information.

We have tried to emphasize the importance of basic scientific and clinical mechanisms, and common diseases as opposed to rare syndromes. The clinical features and laboratory findings are summarized and illustrated; treatment is briefly outlined.

This book is intended for medical students, but will be useful to anyone who needs a concise and up-to-date introduction to haematology, for example nurses, medical laboratory scientists and those in professions supplementary to medicine.

We particularly wish to thank June Elliott who has patiently word-processed the manuscript through many revisions and Jonathan Rowley and his colleagues at Blackwell Science.

Atul Mehta
Victor Hoffbrand
January 2000

1 Haemopoiesis: physiology and pathology

Definition and sites

Haemopoiesis is the process whereby blood cells are made (Fig. 1.1). The yolk sac, and later the liver and spleen, are important in fetal life but after birth normal haemopoiesis is restricted to the bone marrow. Infants have haemopoietic marrow in all bones but in adults it is in the central skeleton and proximal ends of long bones (normal fat to haemopoietic tissue ratio of about 50:50) (Fig. 1.4b). Expansion of haemopoiesis down the long bones may occur, e.g. in leukaemias and chronic haemolytic anaemias. The liver and spleen can resume extramedullary haemopoiesis when there is marrow replacement, e.g. in myelofibrosis, or excessive demand, e.g. in severe haemolytic anaemias.

Stem cell and progenitor cells

A common primitive stem cell in the marrow has the capacity to self replicate, proliferate and differentiate to increasingly specialized progenitor cells which, after many cell divisions within the marrow, form mature cells (red cells, granulocytes, monocytes, platelets and lymphocytes) of the peripheral blood (Fig. 1.2). The earliest recognizable red cell precursor is a pronormoblast and the earliest recognizable granulocyte or monocyte precursor is a myeloblast. An early lineage division is between progenitors for lymphoid and myeloid cells. Stem and progenitor cells cannot be recognized morphologically; they resemble lymphocytes. Progenitor cells can be detected by special *in vitro* assays in which they form colonies (e.g. colony forming units for granulocytes and monocytes, CFU-GM, or for red cells, BFU-E and CFU-E). Stem and progenitor cells also circulate in the peripheral blood. The stromal cells of the marrow (fibroblasts, endothelial cells, macrophages, fat cells) have adhesion molecules which react with corresponding ligands on the stem cells and maintain their viability.

Growth factors

Haemopoiesis is regulated by growth factors (GFs) (Table 1.1) which usually act in synergy with each other. These are glycoproteins produced by stromal cells, T lymphocytes, the liver and, for erythropoietin, the kidney. While some GFs act mainly on receptors on the surface of primitive cells, others act on later cells already committed to a particular lineage. They also affect the function of mature cells. Growth factors inhibit apoptosis (programmed cell death) of their target cells. Growth factors in clinical use include erythropoietin (EPO), granulocyte colony-stimulating factor (G-CSF), granulocyte-macrophage colony-stimulating factor (GM-CSF). Thrombopoietin is under trial.

Signal transduction

The binding of a GF with its surface receptor on the haemopoietic cell activates a complex series of biochemical reactions by which a message is transmitted into the nucleus (Fig. 1.3). The pathways involve sequential phosphorylation of substrates by protein kinases. The signal activates transcription factors which in turn activate or inhibit gene transcription. The signal may activate pathways which cause the cell to enter cell cycle (replicate), differentiate, maintain viability (inhibition of apoptosis) or become functionally active (e.g. enhancement of cell killing by neutrophils).

Assessment of haemopoiesis

Haemopoiesis can be assessed clinically by performing a full blood count on peripheral blood (see Table 3.1). Bone marrow aspiration also allows assessment of the later stages of maturation of haemopoietic cells (Fig. 1.4a–f; see Chapter 7 for indications). Trephine biopsy provides a core of bone and bone marrow to show architecture.

Table 1.1 Haemopoietic growth factors.

Act on stromal cells
IL-1 ⎱ Stimulate production of GM-CSF, G-CSF, M-CSF, IL-6   TNF ⎰
Act on pluripotential cells
Stem cell factor
Act on early multipotential cells
IL-3   IL-4   IL-6   GM-CSF
Act on committed progenitor cells*
G-CSF   M-CSF   IL-5 (eosinophil CSF)   Erythropoietin   Thrombopoietin

*These growth factors (especially G-CSF and thrombopoietin) also act on earlier cells.
G-CSF, granulocyte colony-stimulating factor; GM-CSF, granulocyte-macrophage colony-stimulating factor; IL, interleukin; M-CSF, monocyte colony stimulating factor.

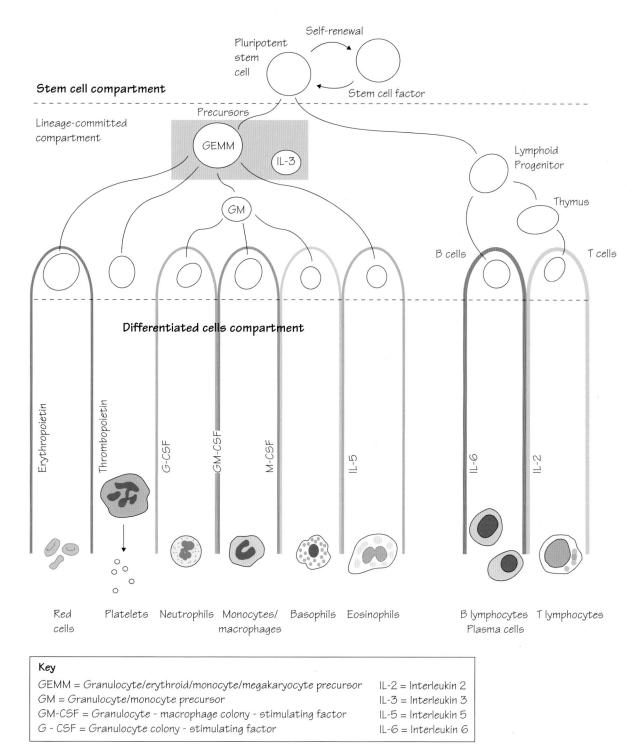

Self-renewal

Pluripotent stem cell

Stem cell factor

Stem cell compartment

Lineage-committed compartment

Precursors

GEMM

IL-3

Lymphoid Progenitor

Thymus

B cells

T cells

GM

Differentiated cells compartment

Erythropoietin

Thrombopoietin

G-CSF

GM-CSF

M-CSF

IL-5

IL-6

IL-2

Red cells

Platelets

Neutrophils

Monocytes/ macrophages

Basophils

Eosinophils

B lymphocytes Plasma cells

T lymphocytes

Key

GEMM = Granulocyte/erythroid/monocyte/megakaryocyte precursor
GM = Granulocyte/monocyte precursor
GM-CSF = Granulocyte - macrophage colony - stimulating factor
G - CSF = Granulocyte colony - stimulating factor

IL-2 = Interleukin 2
IL-3 = Interleukin 3
IL-5 = Interleukin 5
IL-6 = Interleukin 6

Fig. 1.1 Haemopoiesis. Showing site of action of growth factors.

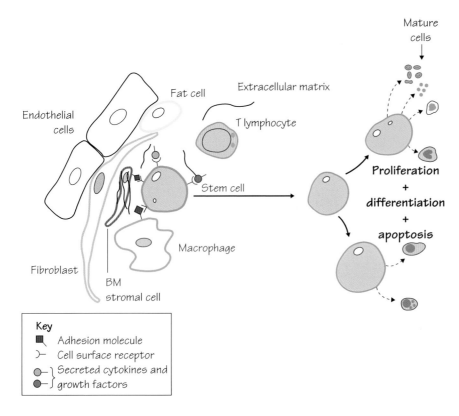

Key
■ Adhesion molecule
)— Cell surface receptor
●—⎫
●—⎬ Secreted cytokines and
      growth factors

Fig. 1.2 Haemopoiesis occurs within the bone marrow microenvironment where haemopoietic stem cells are brought into contact with a range of other cell types. Cell–cell communication is by binding, via cell surface receptors, to adhesion molecules and to fixed or secreted cytokines and growth factors. This binding triggers signal transduction which regulates gene transcription leading to proliferation, differentiation and apoptosis.

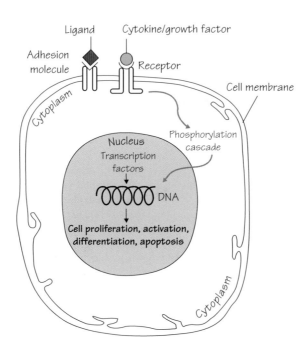

Fig. 1.3 Control of haemopoiesis. Binding of appropriate ligands to surface adhesion molecules or cytokines/growth factors to cell surface receptors induces conformational change (signal transduction) and generation of a cascade of phosphorylation of different proteins. This results in activation of transcription factors which act on DNA to regulate expression of genes affecting cellular proliferation, differentiation, survival and function.

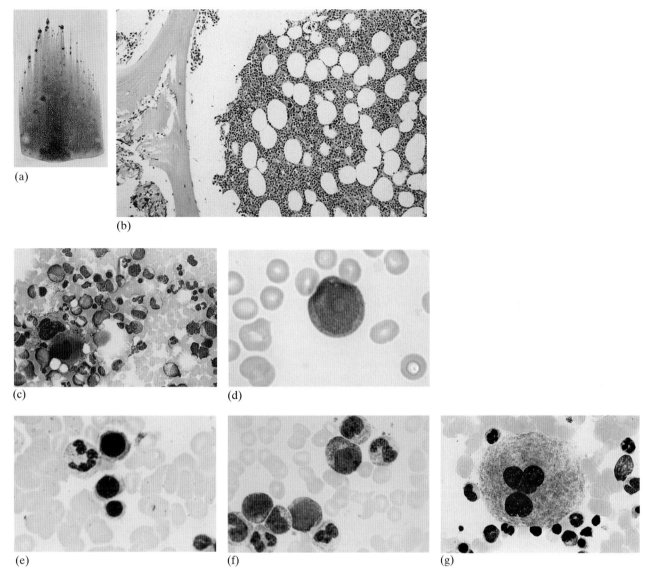

(a)

(b)

(c)

(d)

(e)

(f)

(g)

Fig. 1.4 Normal bone marrow (MGG (May Grunewald Giemsa) stain). (a) Aspirated bone marrow is spread onto a slide, stained and then examined microscopically. (b) Low-power view of a bone marrow trephine biopsy from the iliac crest, showing bone tuberculae, fat spaces and aggregates of haemopoietic cells. (c) Low-power view of bone marrow aspirate, showing two multinucleated cells (megakaryocytes), myeloid cells at different stages of maturation, nucleated cells and mature red cells. Normal marrow has a myeloid/erythroid (M/E) ratio of 2:1–11:1. (d) Myeloblasts (high power) with prominent nucleolus and primary granules. Myeloid cells undergo a total of 12–14 divisions up to promyelocyte stage, after which they mature but no longer divide. (e) A neutrophil with three late normoblasts (high power). Erythroid cells also undergo 12–15 divisions, up to late normoblast stage. (f) As myeloid cells mature, they progress from promyelocyte stage to lose their nucleolus, develop secondary granules and become myelocytes. The nucleus becomes smaller (metamyelocyte) and finally segments (neutrophil). (g) Megakaryocyte (high power). The nucleus segments to give 2, 4, 8, 16, 32 and finally up to 64 segments. Segments of cytoplasm break off to give rise to platelets.

Normal blood cells I: Red cells and platelets

Peripheral blood cells

Normal peripheral blood contains mainly mature cells which do not undergo further division.

Red cells (erythrocytes)

Red cells contain haemoglobin (Hb) which allows them to carry oxygen (O_2) and carbon dioxide (CO_2). Haemoglobin is composed of four polypeptide globin chains each with an iron containing haem molecule (Fig. 2.1). Embryonic haemoglobins (Portland, Gower I and II) are present in early fetal life, fetal haemoglobin (Hb F) dominates by late fetal life (Table 2.1). A switch occurs at 3–6 months in the neonatal period to normal adult haemoglobin (Hb A) (Fig. 2.2). The ability of haemoglobin to bind O_2 is measured as the haemoglobin–O_2 dissociation curve. Raised concentrations of 2,3-DPG, H^+ ions or CO_2 decrease O_2 affinity, allowing more O_2 delivery to tissues (Fig. 2.3). Hb F has a higher, and sickle Hb (Hb S) a lower O_2 affinity than Hb A. **Erythropoietin** controls the production of red cells. It is produced in the peritubular complex of the kidney (90%), liver and other organs. Erythropoietin stimulates mixed lineage and red cell progenitors as well as pronormoblasts and early erythroblasts to proliferate, differentiate and produce haemoglobin (Table 2.1). Erythropoietin secretion is stimulated by reduced O_2 supply to the kidney receptor (see Chapter 27, Table 27.1).

The glycolytic pathway (Fig. 2.4) is the main source of energy (ATP) required to maintain red cell shape and deformability. The *hexose monophosphate* 'shunt' pathway provides the main source of reduced nicotinamide adenine dinucleotide phosphate (NADPH), which maintains reduced glutathione (GSH) and protects haemoglobin and the membrane proteins against oxidant damage. Mature red cells have no nucleus, ribosomes or mitochondria. They survive for about 120 days and are removed by macrophages of the reticuloendothelial system (Chapter 4).

The red cell membrane (Fig. 2.5) is a bipolar lipid layer which anchors surface antigens. It has a protein skeleton (spectrin, actin, protein 4.1 and ankyrin) which maintains the red cell's biconcave shape and deformability.

Developing red cells in the marrow (erythroblasts) are nucleated (see Fig. 1.4); the nucleus condenses with maturation, to be extruded prior to red cell release into the circulation. **Reticulocytes** (Fig. 2.6) are young non-nucleated red cells which retain RNA (stainable by supravital stains). They increase in number following acute haemorrhage, treatment of haematinic deficiency and in haemolytic anaemias. Ten to fifteen percent of developing erythroblasts die within the marrow without producing mature red cells. This 'ineffective erythropoiesis' is increased in, for example, thalassaemia major, myelofibrosis and megaloblastic anaemia.

Platelets
Thrombopoiesis

Megakaryocytes (see Fig. 1.4g) are large multinucleated cells derived from haemopoietic stem cells in the bone

Table 2.1 Normal haemoglobins.

	Hb A	Hb A$_2$	Hb F
Structure	$\alpha_2\beta_2$	$\alpha_2\delta_2$	$\alpha_2\gamma_2$
Normal adult (%)	96–98	1.5–3.5	0.5–0.8

Embryonic haemoglobins

Portland
Gower I
Gower II

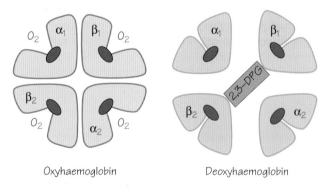

Oxyhaemoglobin   Deoxyhaemoglobin

Fig. 2.1 Normal adult haemoglobin contains four globin (polypeptide) chains ($\alpha_1 \alpha_2, \beta_1 \beta_2$), each with its own haem molecule. These chains undergo conformational change and move with respect to each other when binding O_2 and CO_2. 2,3 diphosphoglycerate (2,3-DPG) binds between the β chains to reduce affinity for O_2 and allow O_2 release to the tissues.

Table 2.2 Haematinics.

Serum iron	10–30 µmol/L
Total iron binding capacity	40–75 µmol/L (2–4 g/L as transferrin)
Serum ferritin	40–340 µg/L (males)
	15–150 µg/L (females)
Serum folate	3.0–15.0 µg/L (4–30 nmol/L)
Red cell folate	160–640 µg/L (360–1460 nmol/L)
Serum vitamin B$_{12}$	160–925 µg/L (120–682 pmol/L)

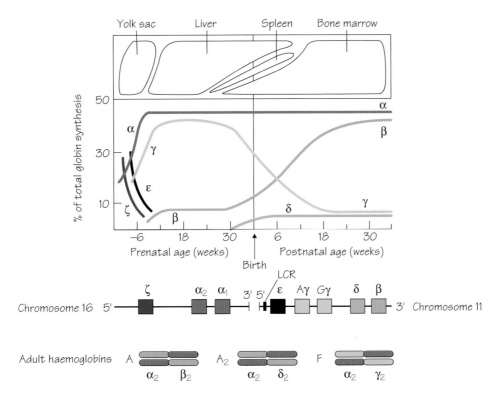

Fig. 2.2 The globin genes are located on chromosomes 16 (ζ, α) and 11 (ε, Gγ, Aγ, δ, β). A 5′ locus control region (LCR) is important in regulating γ and β globin gene expression. Different genes are transcribed during pre- and postnatal life, and the chains are synthesized independently and then combine to produce the different haemoglobins. The γ genes differ to produce either a glutamic acid (Gγ) or alanine (Aγ) residue at position 136. Whereas haemopoiesis occurs in yolk sac, liver and spleen prenatally, it is confined to marrow postnatally.

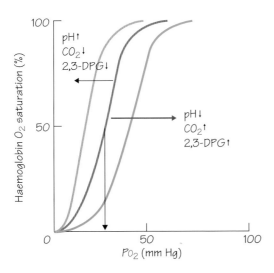

Fig. 2.3 The p50 is the partial pressure of oxygen at which haemoglobin is 50% saturated (red curve, normally 27 mmHg). Decreased oxygen affinity, with increasing p50 (green curve) occurs as carbon dioxide concentration increases or pH decreases (Bohr effect) or 2,3-DPG levels rise. Increased oxygen affinity occurs during the opposite circumstances or may be a characteristic of a variant haemoglobin, which may lead to polycythaemia (see Chapter 27), e.g. Hb Chesapeake or Hb F.

marrow. Platelets break off from the megakaryocyte cytoplasm and enter the peripheral blood. Thrombopoietin is a hormone produced mainly in the liver which stimulates megakaryocyte and platelet production. Both thrombopoietin and erythropoietin have some action on mixed lineage progenitors so that although their predominant action is on platelets and red cells, respectively, they also have some stimulatory action on both lineages. Thrombopoietin increases platelet production by increasing differentiation of stem cells into megakaryocytes, increasing megakaryocyte numbers and also by increasing the number of divisions undertaken by megakaryocyte nuclei (ploidy). Platelets (Fig. 2.7) are non-nucleated cells required for normal haemostasis (see Chapter 28). They circulate for 7–10 days and are then destroyed in the spleen or the pulmonary vascular bed. Their lifespan is reduced when there is increased platelet consumption (thrombosis, infection and splenic enlargement). Platelets appear in peripheral blood films as granular basophilic forms with a mean diameter of 1–2 μm. The normal concentration is 140–400 × 10^9/L; a lower number is found in neonates (100–300 × 10^9/L) and among certain racial populations, e.g. in Southern Europe or the Middle East.

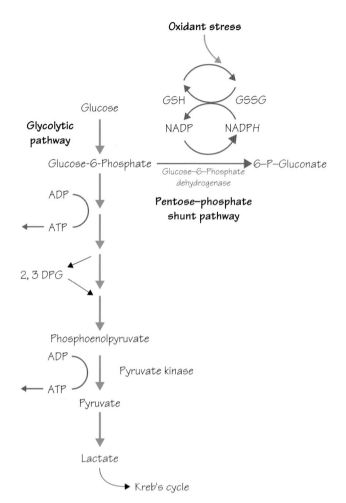

Fig. 2.4 Red cell metabolism.

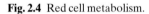

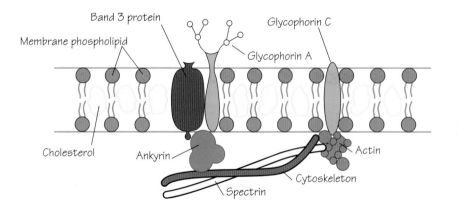

Fig. 2.6 Reticulocyte (brilliant cresyl blue stain) with blue strands of RNA.

Fig. 2.5 The red cell membrane consists of fat (a phospholipid bilayer and cholesterol), carbohydrate and proteins. The proteins are either integral and transmembrane (e.g. band 3, glycophorin) or extrinsic and cytoskeletal (e.g. spectrin, actin, ankyrin) and they maintain red cell shape and anchor red cell antigens.

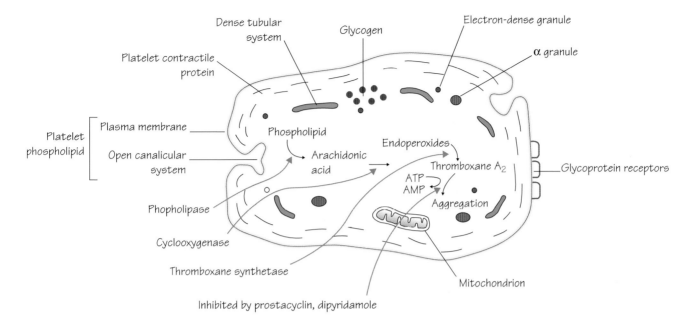

Fig. 2.7 Diagram of a platelet. Platelets do not have nuclei. Electron dense granules contain platelet nucleotides (ADP), Ca^{2+} and serotonin. α granules contain a heparin antagonist (platelet factor 4), platelet derived growth factor, β thromboglobulin, fibrinogen and other clotting factors. Glycoproteins on the surface, e.g. Ia (adhesion to collagen), Ib (defective in Bernard–Soulier syndrome) and IIb/IIIa (defective in thrombasthenia) are important in adhesion and aggregation. The plasma membrane and canalicular system provides a large reactive surface on which plasma coagulation factors are absorbed and activated. Aspirin and sulphinpyrazone inhibit platelet function by inhibiting cyclo-oxygenase. Prostacyclin from endothelial cells and dipyridamole inhibit the action of thromboxane A_2.

3 Normal blood cells II: Granulocytes

Granulocyte and monocyte production occurs in the bone marrow and is controlled by growth factors (see Table 1.1). External stimuli (e.g. infection, fever, inflammation, allergy, trauma) act on cytokine networks to increase production of these growth factors. The cytokines interleukin-1 and tumour necrosis factor (TNF) form part of this complex network. The earliest recognizable granulocyte precursors in the marrow are promyelocytes. These undergo further division and maturation into myelocytes, metamyelocytes and, finally, granulocytes (neutrophils, eosinophils and basophils). Primary granules, present in promyelocytes, contain lysosomal enzymes (e.g. peroxidase, hydrolases). Secondary granules containing enzymes (peroxidase, lysosyme, alkaline phosphatase and lactoferrin) appear later. Basophil granules also contain histamine and heparin.

Function of white cells

The primary function of white cells is to protect the body against infection. They work closely with protein components of the immune response, immunoglobulins and complement. They also produce cytokines which augment function or stimulate proliferation of other cells. Neutrophils, eosinophils, basophils and monocytes are all phagocytes; they ingest and destroy pathogens and cell debris. Phagocytes are attracted to bacteria at the site of inflammation by chemotactic substances released from damaged tissues or by complement components. Opsonization is the coating of cells or foreign particles by immunoglobulin or complement; this aids phagocytosis (engulfment) because phagocytes have Fc and C3b (see below) receptors. Killing involves reduction of pH within the phagocytic vacuole, the release of granule contents and the production of antimicrobial oxidants and superoxides (the 'respiratory burst').

Neutrophils

Neutrophils (polymorphs) (Fig. 3.1a) are usually the most numerous mature peripheral blood leucocyte. They have a short lifespan of around 10h in the circulation (circulating pool). About 50% of neutrophils in peripheral blood are attached to the walls of blood vessels (marginating pool). They enter tissues by migrating in response to chemotactic factors. Their mobility results from the presence of adhesion molecules on their surface which interact with the vascular endothelium. Migration, phagocytosis and killing are energy-dependent functions. Neutrophil function tests separately assess chemotaxis/migration, phagocytosis,

Table 3.1 Normal peripheral blood count.

Cell	Normal concentration
Haemoglobin	11.5–15.5 g/dL (female)
	13.5–17.5 g/dL (male)
Red cell	3.9–5.6×10^{12}/L (female)
	4.5–6.5×10^{12}/L (male)
Reticulocyte	0.5–3.5%
	approx. 25–95×10^9/L
White cells	4.0–11.0×10^9/L
Neutrophils	2.5–7.5×10^9/L
	(1.5–7.5×10^9/L in black people)
Eosinophils	0.04–0.4×10^9/L
Basophils	0.01–0.1×10^9/L
Monocytes	0.2–0.8×10^9/L
Lymphocytes	1.5–3.0×10^9/L
Haematocrit	0.38–0.54
Mean cell volume	80–100 fl
Mean cell haemoglobin	27–33

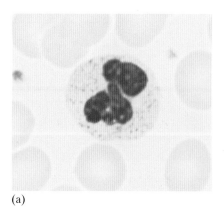
(a)

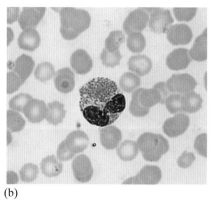
(b)

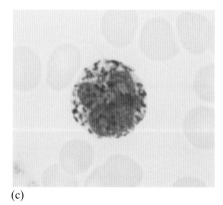
(c)

Fig. 3.1 Normal peripheral blood cells (MGG): (a) neutrophil; (b) eosinophil; (c) basophil.

degranulation and the metabolic process involved in killing. The concentration in the blood may be lower in certain racial populations, e.g. Negro.

Eosinophils

Eosinophils have similar kinetics of production, differentiation and circulation to neutrophils; the growth factor IL-5 is important in regulating their production. They have a characteristic bi-lobed nucleus (Fig. 3.1b) and red-orange staining granules. They are particularly important in the response to parasitic and allergic diseases. Release of their granule contents onto larger pathogens (e.g. helminths) allows their destruction and subsequent phagocytosis. Histamine is an important component of their granules.

Basophils

Basophils are related to small darkly staining cells in the bone marrow and tissues (mast cells) and both are derived from granulocyte precursors in the bone marrow. They are the least numerous of peripheral blood leucocytes and have characteristic large dark purple granules which may obscure the nucleus (Fig. 3.1c). The granule contents include histamine and heparin and are released following binding of IgE to surface receptors. They play an important part in immediate hypersensitivity reactions. Mast cells also have an important role in defence against allergens and parasitic pathogens.

4 Normal blood cells III: Monocytes and the reticuloendothelial system

Monocytes

Monocytes (Fig. 4.1) circulate for 20–40h and then enter tissues as tissue macrophages where they mature and carry out their principal functions. Within tissues they survive for many days, possibly months. They have variable morphology in peripheral blood, but are mononuclear, have greyish cytoplasm with vacuoles and small granules. Within tissues, they often have long cytoplasmic projections allowing them to communicate widely with other cells.

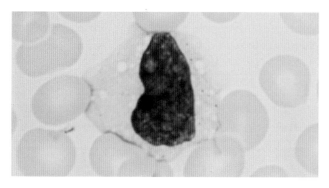

Fig. 4.1 Normal monocyte.

Reticuloendothelial system

This is used to describe monocyte derived cells (Fig. 4.2) which are distributed throughout the body in multiple organs and tissues. The system includes Kupffer's cells in the liver, alveolar macrophages in the lung, mesangial cells in the kidney, microglial cells in the brain and macrophages within the bone marrow, spleen, lymph nodes, skin and serosal surfaces. The principal functions of the reticuloendothelial system are to:

• phagocytose and destroy pathogens and cellular debris;

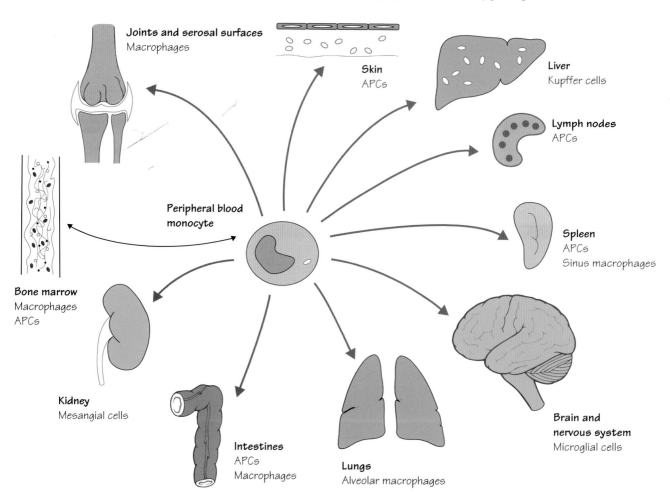

Fig. 4.2 The reticuloendothelial system. APC, antigen presenting cell.

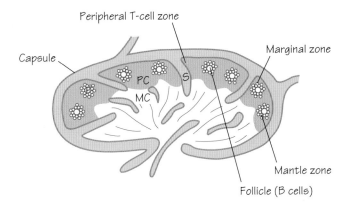

Fig. 4.3 Diagramatic section through a lymph node. The marginal zone is a thin rim around the mantle. F, follicle and germinal centre; MC, medullary cords; PC, paracortex (interfollicular area); S, sinus.

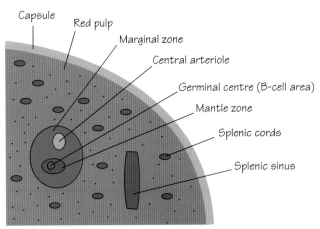

Fig. 4.4 The splenic arterioles are surrounded by a periarteriolar lymphatic sheath — the 'white pulp'. This is composed of T cells, antigen presenting interdigitating cells. Blood flows through the meshwork of the red pulp to find its way into sinuses which are the venous outflow. Part of the splenic blood flow bypasses this filtration process to pass directly through to the veins.

• process and present antigens to lymphoid cells (the antigen presenting cells react principally with T cells with whom they 'interdigitate' in lymph nodes, spleen, thymus, bone marrow and tissues);
• produce cytokines (e.g. IL-1) which regulate and participate within cytokine and growth factor networks governing haemopoiesis, inflammation and cellular responses.

The cells of the reticuloendothelial system (RES) are particularly localized in tissues which may come into contact with external allergens or pathogens. The main organs of the RES allow its cells to communicate with lymphoid cells, and include the liver, spleen, lymph nodes, bone marrow, thymus and intestinal tract associated lymphoid tissue. The anatomy of lymph nodes and spleen are illustrated in Figs 4.3 and 4.4. An additional function of the spleen is to cause blood to be filtered from the arteriolar circulation — the white pulp — through the endothelial meshwork of the red pulp to the sinuses of the venous circulation. This filtration process allows removal of unwanted particulate matter (e.g. opsonized bacteria) as well as removal of effete cells or of unwanted material from within deformable red cells (e.g. nuclear remnants, haemosiderin granules).

5 Normal blood cells IV: Lymphocytes

Lymphocytes are an essential component of the immune response and are derived from haemopoietic stem cells. A common lymphoid stem cell undergoes differentiation and proliferation to give rise to B cells, which mediate humoral or antibody-mediated immunity, and T cells (processed in the thymus), mediating cell-mediated immunity (see Fig. 1.1). Mature lymphocytes appear as small mononuclear cells which have scanty blue cytoplasm (Fig. 5.1). The majority of peripheral blood lymphocytes (70%) are T cells, which typically have more cytoplasm than B cells and may contain granules.

Lymphocyte maturation occurs principally in bone marrow for B cells and in the thymus for T cells but also involves the lymph nodes, liver, spleen and other parts of the reticuloendothelial system. The antigens expressed on the surface of a cell can be recognized in the laboratory by reaction with monoclonal antibody reagents. The cluster of differentiation (CD) nomenclature system has evolved as a means of classifying these antigens. Although most frequently applied to lymphocytes, it is applicable to all haemopoietic cells (see Appendix I). Lymphocytes have the longest lifespan of any leucocyte, and some (e.g. 'memory' B cells) may live for many years.

Immune response

Specificity of the immune response derives from amplification of antigen-selected T and B cells. The T cell receptor (TCR) on T cells and surface membrane immunoglobulin (sIg) on B cells are molecules which have a variable and a constant portion. The variability ensures that a specific antigen is recognized by a lymphocyte with a matching variable region. The genetic mechanisms required to generate the required diversity are common to both T and B cells (Fig. 5.2). They involve rearrangement of variable, joining, diversity and constant region genes to generate genes coding for surface receptors (Ig or TCR) capable of reacting specifically with an enormous array of antigens.

The immune response (Fig. 5.3) involves interaction between T cells, B cells and antigen presenting cells (APCs). Mature T cells are of three main types: helper cells expressing the CD4 antigen; suppressor cells expressing CD8; and cytotoxic cells expressing CD8. Developing T cells are 'educated' in the thymus only to react to foreign antigens, and to develop tolerance to self human leucocyte antigens (HLA). If antigen is presented by an APC alongside the HLA (major histocompatability complex, MHC class II) to a CD4+ T cell, T cell activation and proliferation result. CD8+ cytotoxic cells require the antigen to be presented to them alongside MHC class I molecules. B cells can also interact directly with antigen. Adhesion molecules mediate these cellular interactions. Reaction between antigen and appropriate receptor (sIg or TCR) leads to cellular proliferation and differentiation. This process is augmented by cytokines released by APCs (e.g. IL-6, IL-7) and by interacting T cells (e.g. IL-2) which stimulate T and B cell proliferation. CD8+ suppressor T cells have an important role in regulating B cell proliferation. CD8+ cytotoxic T cells are capable of directly lysing APCs which present appropriate antigen in association with MHC class I molecules.

Natural killer cells

Natural killer cells are neither T nor B cells, though are often CD8+. They characteristically have prominent granules and are often large granular lymphocytes. These cells are not governed by MHC restriction and can kill target cells by direct adhesion. They can also bind to a target cell which has antibody bound to it (antibody-dependent cell-mediated cytotoxicity, ADCC).

Immunoglobulins

These are gammaglobulins produced by plasma cells. There are five main groups: IgG, IgM, IgA, IgD and IgE. Each is composed of light and heavy chains, and each chain is made up of variable, joining and constant regions (Fig. 5.4).

Complement

This is a group of plasma proteins and cell surface receptors which, if activated, interact with cellular and humoral elements in the inflammatory response (Fig. 5.5). The complete molecule is capable of direct lysis of cell membranes and of pathogens sensitized by antibody. The C3b component coats cells making them sensitive to phagocytosis by macrophages. C3a and C5a may also activate chemotaxis by phagocytes and activate mast cells and basophils to release mediators of inflammation.

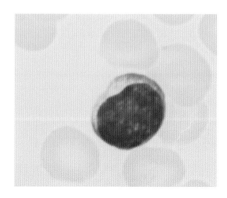

Fig. 5.1 Lymphocyte.

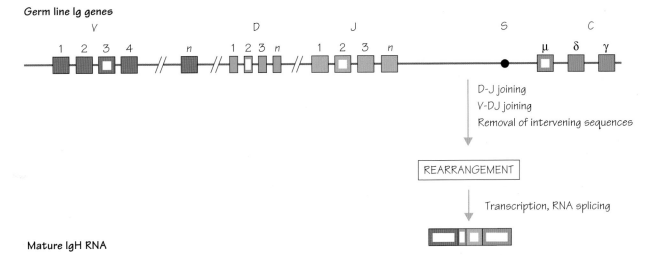

Germa line Ig genes

Mature IgH RNA

Fig. 5.2 Immunoglobulin gene rearrangement and transcription. Immunoglobulin heavy chain genes occur as segments for variable (V), diversity (D), joining (J) and constant (C) regions. The class of the immunoglobulin depends on which of the constant region genes (μ, δ, γ, α, ϵ) is transcribed. The switch region (S) allows switching between classes. Diversity occurs through variability of which V segment joins which D and which J segment; the enzyme terminal deoxynucleotidyl transferase (TdT) randomly inserts new bases into D region DNA to generate additional diversity. Recombinase enzymes join up rearranged segments of DNA and intervening sequences are deleted. Similar rearrangements occur at the immunoglobulin light chain (κ and λ) and T cell receptor (α/β, γ/δ) loci. In the example shown, V_3 joins D_2, J_2 and μ.

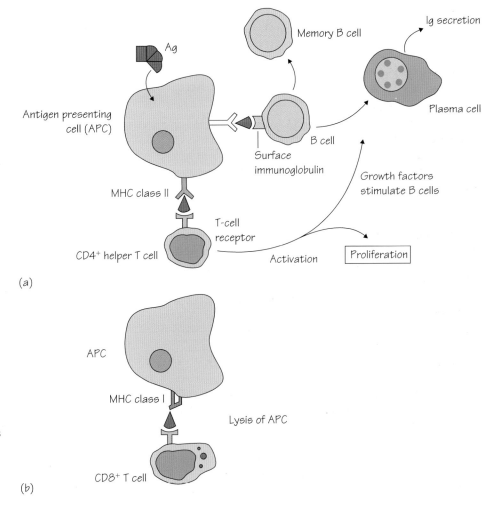

Fig. 5.3 (a) Antigen is phagocytosed and processed by the antigen presenting cell (APC), which is a macrophage. If antigen is presented with the major histocompatibility complex (MHC) class II molecule to a CD4$^+$ (helper) T cell which has an appropriate configuration of its T cell receptor, the T cell will become activated, proliferate and facilitate proliferation of appropriate B cells. B cells also interact with antigen presented by the APC, but to a different epitope. (b) If processed antigen linked to MHC class I molecules is presented to a cytotoxic (CD8$^+$) T cell, it will trigger proliferation of a clone of cytotoxic T cells which will lyse the APC.

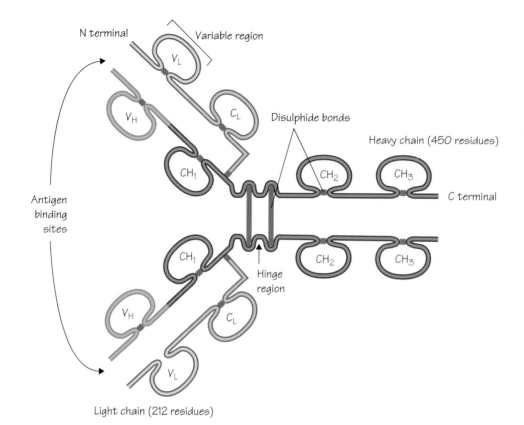

Fig. 5.4 The basic structure of IgG consists of two heavy chains and two light chains, each of which has a variable region (N terminal, antigen binding area) and a relatively constant region (C terminal). The constant portion of the heavy chain is further divided into three structurally discrete regions (CH1, CH2, CH3). The whole structure is stabilized by interchain and intrachain disulphide bonds.

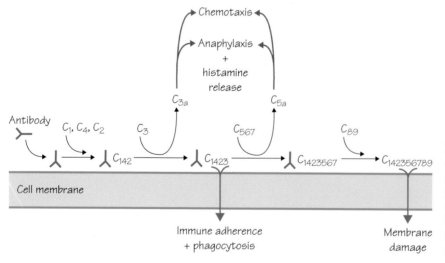

Fig. 5.5 Antibody binding may lead to activation of the complement cascade and generation of mediators of inflammation, phagocytosis and membrane damage. The alternative pathway of complement involves direct activation and amplification of C3 by endotoxin or aggregated immunoglobulin.

History
Anaemia
• Symptoms: shortness of breath on exertion, tiredness, headache or angina, more marked if anaemia is severe, of rapid onset and in older subjects.
• Causes: e.g. bleeding, dietary deficiency, malabsorption, systemic illness, haemolysis, bone marrow failure, inherited abnormalities of red cells.

Leucopenia
• Neutropenia, particularly if neutrophils are $<0.5\times10^9$/L, frequently leads to bacterial or fungal infection in skin, mouth, throat and chest.
• Pus is lacking.
• Lymphopenia predisposes to viral infection (e.g. herpes zoster), tuberculosis.
• Infection is often atypical, caused by organisms non-pathogenic for normal individuals, rapidly progressive and difficult to treat.
• Functional defects of neutrophils and lymphocytes also predispose to infection.

Thrombocytopenia
• Spontaneous bruising (ecchymoses) or petechiae, mucosal bleeding, e.g. epistaxis, menorrhagia. Bleeding following trauma is increased with platelets $<50\times10^9$/L. Spontaneous bleeding occurs when platelets $<10\times10^9$/L.
• Functional platelet defects also predispose to bleeding.

Coagulation factor defects
• Easy bleeding after trauma (e.g. circumcision, dental treatment); spontaneous haemorrhage in deep tissues (e.g. muscles, joints); family history.
• Acquired coagulation defects often accompanied by thrombocytopenia; spontaneous skin bleeding and excessive bleeding in response to trauma.

NB: Combination of anaemia, excessive bleeding and/or infection suggest pancytopenia caused by bone marrow failure (see Chapter 18).

Other symptoms (Fig. 6.1)
• Weight loss, fever, pruritus and skin rash—lymphoma or myeloproliferative disorder.
• Bone pain, symptoms of hypercalcaemia (thirst, polyuria, constipation)—myeloma.
• Left hypochondrial pain—splenomegaly.
• Painless lymphadenopathy.
• Joint pains—gout caused by hyperuricaemia.

Family history
Inherited anaemia (e.g. genetic disorders of haemoglobin), coagulation disorders (e.g. haemophilia) and certain leucocyte disorders.

Drug history
Haemolytic anaemia in G6PD deficiency; disordered platelet function caused by aspirin; drug-induced agranulocytosis; macrocytosis of red cells caused by alcohol.

Operations
Gastrectomy, intestinal resection.

Examination
Includes testing of urine for protein and sugar.
• Pallor of mucous membranes, if Hb<9g/dL.
• Tachycardia, systolic murmur.
• Jaundice (haemolytic or megaloblastic anaemia); pigment (gallstones).
• Lymphadenopathy (generalized or localized) (Table 6.1).
• Skin changes, e.g. purpura caused by thrombocytopenia, vitiligo associated with pernicious anaemia, melanin pigmentation in iron overload, ankle ulcers in haemolytic anaemia, rashes caused by tumour infiltration.
• Nail changes (e.g. koilonychia in iron deficiency).
• Signs of infection (mouth, throat, skin, perineum, chest) associated with neutropenia.
• Mouth, e.g. angular cheilosis in iron deficiency, glossitis in B$_{12}$ or folate deficiency.
• Hepatomegaly or splenomegaly (Table 6.2).

Table 6.1 Causes of lymphadenopathy.

Local

Localized bacterial/viral infection
Skin condition—e.g. trauma, eczema
Malignant—secondary carcinoma, lymphoma

General

Infection
   e.g. bacterial endocarditis, tuberculosis
   Viral—HIV, infectious mononucleosis, cytomegalovirus
   toxoplasmosis
Malignancy
   e.g. lymphoma, lymphoid leukaemias
Inflammatory disorders
   e.g. sarcoidosis, connective tissue diseases
Generalized allergic conditions
   e.g. widespread eczema

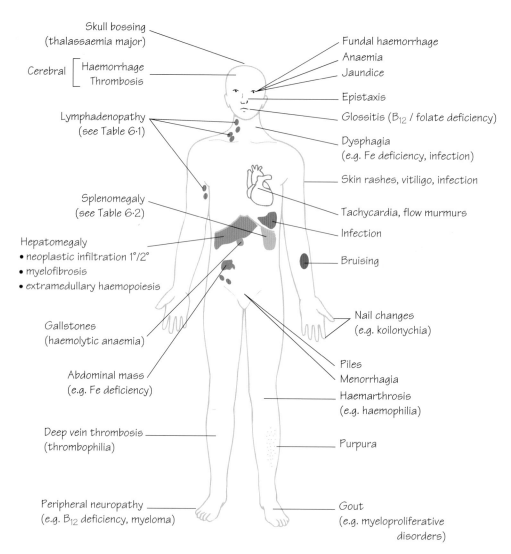

Fig. 6.1 Physical signs in haematological disease.

- Nervous system examination, e.g. B$_{12}$ neuropathy, peripheral neuropathy in myeloma, amyloidosis, malignant infiltration in central nervous system leukaemia.
- Optic fundi, e.g. haemorrhage in severe anaemia, hyperviscosity in polycythaemia.

Special investigations

Haematological diseases are often multisystem disorders and a range of special investigations are frequently required to define the extent and stage of the disease.

Radiological investigations particularly helpful in these patients include:

- X-rays to detect evidence of infection, bone erosion, marrow expansion caused by extramedullary haemopoiesis.
- Ultrasound to confirm presence of abdominal masses, gallstones, detect and assess size of spleen/lymph nodes,

define extent of swellings and detect blood or pus in patients with excessive bleeding or atypical infection, to detect deep vein thrombosis.

- Computed tomography (CT) scan to detect infection (e.g. lungs), lymphadenopathy, abdominal organ enlargement, bleeding and thrombosis.
- Magnetic resonance imaging (MRI) scanning is a sensitive way of detecting bone damage, e.g. in sickle cell anaemia, myeloma or deep soft-tissue lesions.
- Endoscopy often required in the gastrointestinal investigation of iron deficiency anaemia.
- Others, e.g. electrocardiogram (ECG), echocardiogram.

Nuclear medicine studies allow study of organ function, and tests useful to haematologists include the following.

- Isotope labelling of cells followed by scanning, e.g. autologous red cells can be labelled with radioactive chromium/technetium, reinjected and their lifespan measured,

Table 6.2 Causes of splenomegaly.

Haemolytic anaemia

Hereditary spherocytosis, autoimmune haemolytic anaemia, thalassaemia major or intermedia, sickle cell anaemia (before infarction occurs)

Haematological malignancies

Lymphoma, CLL, ALL, AML, CML*
Polycythaemia vera, myelofibrosis*
Myelodysplasia

Storage diseases

Gaucher's*
Amyloid

Liver disease and portal hypertension

Congestive cardiac failure

Infection

Malaria*
Leishmaniasis*
Bacterial endocarditis
Viral infections, e.g. infectious mononucleosis

*Causes of massive splenomegaly.
ALL, acute lymphoblastic leukaemia; AML, acute myeloid leukaemia; CLL, chronic lymphocytic leukaemia; CML, chronic myeloid leukaemia.

loss detected in stools and destruction in liver/spleen detected by surface counting. Labelled white cell (gallium) scans can detect occult infection or lymphoma. Labelled platelet scans can measure platelet lifespan and destruction in liver/spleen can be quantified.
• MUGA scanning to assess ventricular damage (e.g. caused by iron overload, anthracycline drugs).
• Positron emission tomography (PET) measures metabolic activity of tissue and is able to distinguish active tumour (positive) from inactive scar tissue (negative).

Routine tests

Full blood count (FBC) (see Table 3.1)

Blood sample in sequestrene (ethylenediaminetetra-acetate, EDTA) anticoagulant tested by an automated analyser. Analysers provide the following.

- Haemoglobin concentration, haematocrit, red cell count.
- Red cell indices (mean cell volume, MCV; mean cell haemoglobin, MCH) (Table 7.1).
- White cell count.
- Differential white cell count (three-part: neutrophils, lymphocytes, monocytes; or five-part to include eosinophils and basophils). White cells are distinguished by use of biochemical staining reactions, light absorbance and scatter, and internal conductivity.
- Platelet count and size.
- Analysers increasingly provide automated reticulocyte counts, enumerate immature platelets ('platelet reticulocytes') and assess intra-erythrocyte haemoglobinization.

Blood film

Blood film is used to assess red cell size/shape; white cell appearance and differential; abnormal cells; platelet size and morphology; detection of parasites, e.g. malaria.

- The film may suggest a diagnosis, e.g. type of haemolytic anaemia, presence of malaria, leukaemia, myelodysplasia. Reticulocyte count (normal 0.5–3.5%) assesses bone marrow response to anaemia; raised in haemolysis, after haemorrhage, and in response to haematinic therapy.

Table 7.1 Classification of anaemia.

Macrocytic (MCV > 98 fl)
Megaloblastic
Vitamin B_{12} or folate deficiency
Other
See Table 12.2
Normocytic (MCV 78–98 fl)
Most haemolytic anaemias
Secondary anaemias
Mixed cases
Microcytic (MCV < 78 fl; MCH usually also < 27 pg/L)
Iron deficiency
Thalassaemia (α or β)
Other haemoglobin defects
Anaemia of chronic disorders (some cases)
Congenital sideroblastic anaemia (some cases)

MCH, mean cell haemoglobin; MCV, mean cell volume.

- Abnormalities of red cell shape and red cell inclusions are listed on page 29.

Special laboratory tests

Investigations of haemolytic anaemia, haemoglobin disorders, haematinic deficiency, coagulation disorders and malignant diseases are discussed in the relevant chapters.

Erythrocyte sedimentation rate (ESR)

This measures the rate of fall of a column of red cells in plasma in 1 h. It is largely determined by plasma concentrations of proteins, especially fibrinogen and globulins. It is raised in anaemia. Normal range rises with age. A raised ESR is a non-specific indicator of an acute phase response and is of value in monitoring disease activity (e.g. rheumatoid arthritis). A raised ESR occurs in inflammatory disorders, infections, malignancy, myeloma, anaemia and pregnancy. The *plasma viscosity* gives comparable information and is increasingly favoured as it can be easily automated. *C-reactive protein* (CRP) is raised in an acute phase response and is valuable in monitoring this. *Whole blood viscosity* is also influenced by the cell counts, and is therefore raised when the red cell count (erythrocrit), white cells count (leucocrit) or platelet count is grossly raised.

Bone marrow aspiration and trephine biopsy

Bone marrow aspiration is from the posterior iliac crest or sternum; indications are listed in Table 7.2. Aspirated cells and particles of marrow are spread on slides, stained by Romanowsky's stain and for iron (Perls' stain; see Fig. 1.4).

Specialized tests may also be performed (Table 7.3).

Table 7.2 Indications for bone marrow aspiration (and trephine)*.

Unexplained cytopenia*
Anaemia, leucopenia, thrombocytopenia
Suspected marrow infiltration*
Leukaemia, myelodysplasia, lymphoma, myeloproliferative disease, myeloma, carcinoma, storage disorders
Suspected infection
Leishmaniasis, tuberculosis

*Bone marrow trephine is also required for pancytopenia or suspected marrow infiltration.

Sophisticated tests
Flow cytometry
Flow cytometry (Fig. 7.1) is an automated technique whereby a population of cells is incubated with specific monoclonal antibodies which are conjugated to a fluorochrome. The labelled cells are then passed in a fluid stream across a laser light source which allows quantitative analysis of antigen expression on the cell population. The technique is important in leukaemia diagnosis and assessment of residual malignant disease.

Chromosomal analysis
Normal individuals have 46 chromosomes: 44 autosomes (22 from each parent) and two sex chromosomes (46 XY = male, 46 XX = female). Chromosomal analysis is made initially by special stains of cells in division. Loss or gain of whole chromosomes, chromosome breaks and loss, inversion or translocation of a part of a chromosome can be detected. *Fluorescent* in situ *hybridization* is a sensitive technique for detecting chromosome abnormalities (Fig. 7.2) which involves the use of a fluorescent DNA probe which hybridizes selectively to a particular chromosome segment, allowing sensitive detection of deletion, translocation and duplication of that segment.

Table 7.3 Special tests on bone marrow cells.

1 Chromosomes
  Cytogenetics, e.g. diagnosis and classification of leukaemia, myelodysplasia
  Fluorescent *in situ* hybridization (FISH)
2 DNA analysis/polymerase chain reaction (PCR), e.g. diagnosis and classification of leukaemia
  Detection of residual malignant disease
3 Immune phenotype analysis
  Diagnosis and classification of leukaemia, lymphoproliferative diseases
  Detection of residual disease
4 Microbiological cultures, e.g. tuberculosis
5 Cytochemistry—diagnosis of acute leukaemias

DNA abnormalities
DNA abnormalities as a cause of haematological disease may be inherited or acquired (Table 7.4). *Inherited* haematological diseases are most commonly autosomal recessive, requiring an individual to inherit two mutant copies (alleles) of a gene (one from each parent) for expression of the disease (homozygotes). Carriers (heterozygotes) have one normal and one mutant allele and may express minor abnormalities. Autosomal dominant diseases are rarer, and require only one mutant allele for full expression of the disease. Sex-linked diseases arise if the mutant gene is on the X chromosome; males, having only one X chromosome, are affected whereas females are usually carriers. *Acquired* DNA abnormalities are frequently present in clones of malignant cell populations and serve as disease markers and clues to pathogenesis (see Chapter 19).

Molecular techniques
These include:
• Southern blotting (Fig. 7.3) which allows assessment of deletion, rearrangement, inversion or duplication of DNA segments. Single base mutations will only be detected,

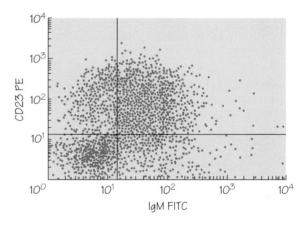

Fig. 7.1 Flow cytometry. Cells are simultaneously tested for expression of CD23 and IgM. The x and y scales indicate the number of cells detected expressing that antigen.

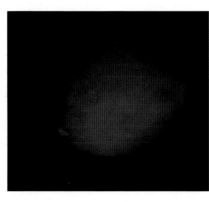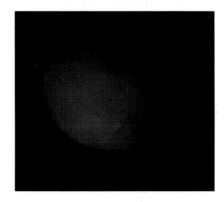

Fig. 7.2 Fluorescent *in situ* hybridization (FISH). Slides have been prepared from a cytogenetic preparation and hybridized with a fluorescent-labelled probe specific for chromosome 7. (a) Normal control showing two signals; (b) a patient with myelodysplasia who has monosomy 7.

Table 7.4 Examples of inherited haematological diseases.

Autosomal recessive

Thalassaemia, sickle cell disease, Gaucher's disease, pyruvate kinase deficiency

Autosomal dominant

Hereditary spherocytosis

Sex-linked

Haemophilia A, haemophilia B, glucose-6-phosphate dehydrogenase (G6PD) deficiency

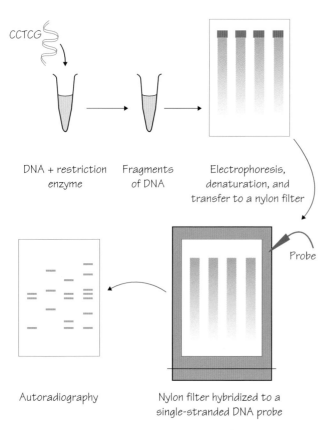

Fig. 7.3 Southern blot technique. Restriction enzymes are bacterial enzymes which recognize specific 3–6 nucleotide sequences (e.g. CCTCG) and cleave DNA whenever that sequence occurs. The fragments of DNA are separated by gel electrophoresis. DNA is then denatured to make it single-stranded and transferred by capillary action to a nylon filter. The filter is then incubated with a single stranded probe, which will hybridize to those DNA fragments with which there is base-pair homology. The Northern blot technique is a way of analysing RNA species by probe hybridization.

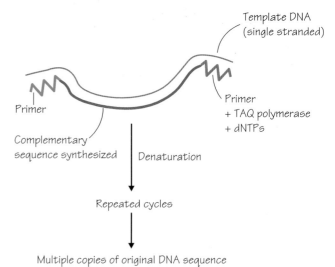

Fig. 7.4 The polymerase chain reaction (PCR) can be used to amplify a DNA segment (typically 0.1–2 kb). The template DNA is denatured and incubated with oligonucleotides (15–20 bp which hybridize specifically to sequences in template DNA and not anywhere else in the genome). The enzyme TAQ polymerase, in the presence of deoxynucleotides (dNTP), allows formation of a complete DNA chain complementary to the template sequence. This process is repeated 40 or so times. Modifications include amplifying a mRNA sequence into DNA and using nucleotides which only bind to a mutant and not a wild type DNA sequence so that only mutant sequences are amplified.

however, if they alter the recognition sequence of a restriction enzyme.
• Polymerase chain reaction (PCR) (Fig. 7.4) can be used to amplify a DNA segment which can then be sequenced or fractionated by size using gel electrophoresis. PCR can also be used to selectively amplify a particular sequence which may, for example, characterize a clone of malignant cells (minimal residual disease, see Chapter 19).
• Gene expression is studied by analysing RNA extracted from fresh cells e.g. by gel electrophoresis (Northern blot). It can be semi-quantitated by using the enzyme reverse transcriptase to generate a DNA copy and then applying a modified PCR technique.

Suspected disorders of haemostasis

Initial screening is with platelet count, prothrombin time (PT), activated partial thromboplastin time (APTT) and thrombin time (TT). These simple tests of the coagulation pathway are performed by automated machines (coagulometers). If a defect of platelet function is suspected, test bleeding time and platelet function. If disseminated intravascular coagulation (DIC) is considered, measure fibrinogen level and test for fibrin degradation products. If a coagulation factor defect is suspected, assay specific clotting factors. A thrombophilia screen may be needed for patients with, or a family history of, thrombosis (see Chapter 32).

Red cell abnormalities

Red cell abnormalities	Causes
Normal	
Macrocyte	Liver disease, alcoholism. Oval in megaloblastic anaemia
Target cell	Iron deficiency, liver disease, haemoglobinopathies, post-splenectomy
Stomatocyte	Liver disease, alcoholism
Pencil cell	Iron deficiency
Ecchinocyte	Liver disease, post-splenectomy
Acanthocyte	Liver disease, abetalipoprotein-aemia, renal failure
Sickle cell	Sickle cell anaemia
Microcyte	Iron deficiency, haemoglobinopathy

Red cell abnormalities	Causes
Spherocyte	Hereditary spherocytosis autoimmune haemolytic anaemia, septicaemia
Fragments	DIC, microangiopathy, HUS, TTP, burns, cardiac valves
Elliptocyte	Hereditary elliptocytosis
Tear drop poikilocyte	Myelofibrosis, extramedullary haemopoiesis
Basket cell	Oxidant damage—e.g. G6PD deficiency, unstable haemoglobin
Howell–Jolly body	Hyposplenism, post-splenectomy
Basophilic stippling	Haemoglobinopathy, lead poisoning, myelodysplasia, haemolytic anaemia
Malarial parasite	Malaria. Other intra-erythrocytic parasites include *Bartonella bacilliformis*, babesiosis
Siderotic granules (Pappenheimer bodies)	Disordered iron metabolism e.g. sideroblastic anaemia, post-splenectomy

8 Benign disorders of white cells: granulocytes, monocytes, macrophages and lymphocytes

Granulocytes and monocytes

Inflammation commonly causes a neutrophil leucocytosis (neutrophilia) (Table 8.1). In addition, neutrophil granules may stain intensely (toxic granulation) and Doehle bodies (cytoplasmic RNA) may be present. A leukaemoid reaction is a profound reactive neutrophilia in which granulocyte precursors (e.g. myelocytes) also appear in the blood. Neutropenia (reduced number of circulating neutrophils; Table 8.2) increases susceptibility to infection, particularly bacterial. The normal neutrophil count is lower in black and Middle Eastern subjects than white people; this has no clinical consequences. Causes of **eosinophilia** are listed in Table 8.3. **Basophilia** (increase in blood basophils to $>0.1 \times 10^9$/L) is uncommon but occurs in myeloproliferative disorders. **Monocytosis** (increase in circulating monocytes to $>1.0 \times 10^9$/L) may occur in chronic infections (bacterial and protozoal, particularly in patients who cannot mount a neutrophil response), in malignancy and in myelodysplasia (see Chapter 21). **Disorders of neutrophil function** may be congenital or acquired and affect neutrophil interaction with immunoglobulin/complement, migration, phagocytosis and microbicidal activity. *Chronic granulomatous disease* is a rare inherited (X-linked) condition in which the cells are able to phagocytose but not kill. Acquired defects occur more commonly for example in diabetes, myelodysplasia and corticosteroid therapy.

Lysosomal storage disease

Hereditary deficiencies of enzymes required for glycolipid metabolism lead to the accumulation of ceramide components in various cells and tissues. *Gaucher's disease* is the most common (autosomal recessive) and is caused by mutations in the gene encoding glucocerebrosidase. Type I (most common) occurs especially among Ashkenazic Jews (age of presentation from infancy to middle age) and does not involve the central nervous system (CNS); types II and III are rarer and do involve the CNS. Clinical and haematological features result from accumulation of Gaucher's cells (Fig. 8.1) in the spleen, liver, skeleton, marrow and in types II and III in the CNS. Treatment is principally by enzyme replacement therapy.

Histiocyte disorders

Histiocytes are the terminally differentiated cells of the monocyte macrophage system and are widely distributed throughout all tissues. Langerhans' cells are macrophages present in epidermis, spleen, thymus, bone, lymph nodes and mucosal surfaces. *Langerhans' cell histiocytosis* (LCH) is a rare single organ or system or multisystem disease

Table 8.1 Causes of neutrophilia (neutrophils $>7.5 \times 10^9$/L).

Bacterial infections
Inflammation, e.g. collagen diseases, Crohn's disease
Trauma/surgery
Tissue necrosis/infarction
Neoplasia
Haemorrhage and haemolysis
Metabolic, e.g. diabetic ketoacidosis
Myeloproliferative disorders
Pregnancy
Drugs, e.g. steriods, GCSF

GCSF, granulocyte colony-stimulating factor.

Table 8.2 Causes of neutropenia (neutrophils $<1.5 \times 10^9$/L). Normal black and Middle Eastern subjects have lower counts.

1 Decreased production

(a) General bone marrow failure, e.g. aplastic anaemia, megaloblastic anaemia, myelodysplasia, acute leukaemia, chemotherapy, replacement by tumour (see Chapter 18)
(b) Specific failure of neutrophil production
    Congenital, e.g. Kostman's syndrome
    Cyclical
    Drug-induced, e.g. sulphonamides, chlorpromazine, clozaril, diuretics, neomercazole, gold

2 Increased destruction

(a) General, e.g. hypersplenism
(b) Specific, e.g. autoimmune—alone or in association with connective tissue disorder, rheumatoid arthritis (Felty's syndrome)

Table 8.3 Causes of eosinophilia (eosinophils $>0.4 \times 10^9$/L).

Allergic diseases, e.g. asthma, hay fever, eczema, pulmonary hypersensitivity reaction (e.g. Loeffler's syndrome)
Parasitic disease
Skin diseases, e.g. psoriasis, drug rash
Drug sensitivity
Connective tissue disease
Haematological malignancy (e.g. Hodgkin lymphoma)
Idiopathic hypereosinophilia
Eosinophilic leukaemia (rare)

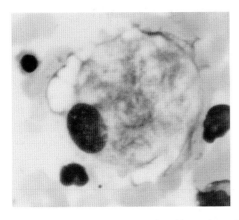

Fig. 8.1 Histiocyte laden with glucocerebroside to give a fibrillar cytoplasmic pattern (Gaucher's cell).

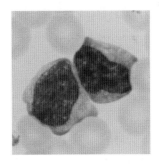

Fig. 8.2 Peripheral blood lymphocytes (activated T cells) in infectious mononucleosis.

occurring principally in childhood (<10 years), with an incidence of 2–5 cases/million population. Clinical features include skin rash, bone pain/swelling, lymphadenopathy, hepatosplenomegaly, endocrine changes (e.g. diabetes insipidus as a result of posterior pituitary involvement). Malignant histiocyte disorders include monocytic variants of acute leukaemia (see Chapter 22) and some types of non-Hodgkin lymphoma (see Chapter 26).

Haemophagocytic syndromes

In these syndromes the bone marrow shows increased numbers of histiocytes which contain ingested blood cells, leading to pancytopenia. The mechanism is poorly understood and prognosis is usually poor. Causes include infection (viral, bacterial, tuberculous), especially in an immunosuppressed host, tumours (e.g. lymphoma) (see Fig. 36.1) or a rare familial type.

Lymphocyte disorders

Lymphocytosis occurs in viral infections, some bacterial infections (e.g. pertussis) and in lymphoid neoplasia.

Lymphopenia (reduction in circulating lymphocytes to <1.5×10⁹/L) occurs in viral infection (e.g. HIV), lymphoma, connective tissue disease, and severe bone marrow failure.

Infectious mononucleosis (*glandular fever*) is caused by Epstein–Barr virus (EBV) infection of B lymphocytes. Atypical circulating lymphocytes are reactive T cells. Cytomegalovirus, other viruses and toxoplasma infections cause a similar blood picture (Fig. 8.2). Clinical features include onset usually in young adults (age 15–40 years), sore throat, lymphadenopathy, fever, morbilliform rash—particularly following treatment with amoxicillin—and jaundice, hepatomegaly and tender splenomegaly in a minority. Complications include autoimmune thrombocytopenia and/or haemolytic anaemia, myocarditis, encephalitis, hepatitis and postviral fatigue syndrome. The Paul–Bunnell test, modified as the monospot slide test, detects heterophile antibodies (antibodies against cells of a different species). These agglutinate sheep red blood cells and, unlike those present in normal people, are not absorbed by guinea-pig kidney cells but are absorbed by ox red blood cells. The test is positive from 1 week after infection and persists for up to 2 months. Viral culture from sputum/saliva and specific IgM and IgG antibody tests against EBV nuclear and capsular antigens are sometimes useful in diagnosis.

Immunodeficiency

Depressed humoral immunity may be congenital (e.g. X-linked agammaglobulinaemia) or acquired (e.g. myeloma and chronic lymphocytic leukaemia (CLL)) and characteristically leads to recurrent pyogenic bacterial infections. Depressed cell mediated immunity may be congenital (e.g. Di George's syndrome) or acquired (e.g. HIV infection, lymphoma, CLL) and causes susceptibility to viral, protozoal and fungal infections, anergy and a secondary defect in humoral immunity. Mixed B and T cell deficiency is common.

HIV infection and AIDS

HIV-1 is a retrovirus transmitted by semen, blood and other body fluids, which infects and kills CD4+ T lymphocytes to cause immune suppression. A non-specific febrile illness with lymphadenopathy often marks initial infection. A proportion of patients progress to AIDS with a CD4 count <0.2×10⁹/L. Clinical manifestations include recurring infections, anaemia and lymphadenopathy. There is an increased risk of non-Hodgkin lymphoma and of Kaposi's sarcoma. Treatment may also induce anaemia; e.g. azidothymidine (AZT) and co-trimoxazole both cause megaloblastic change. Thrombocytopenia, lymphopenia and neutropenia (immune or caused by marrow failure or drug therapy) are also frequent. The bone marrow is usually normo- or hyper-cellular, with dysplastic features and an increase in plasma cells.

9 Iron I: Physiology and deficiency

Distribution of body iron

Iron is contained in haemoglobin, the reticuloendothelial system (RES) (as ferritin and haemosiderin), muscle (myoglobin), plasma (bound to transferrin) and cellular enzymes (e.g. cytochromes, catalase) (Fig. 9.1). Reticuloendothelial cells (macrophages) gain iron from the haemoglobin of effete red cells and release it to plasma transferrin which transports iron to bone marrow and other tissues with transferrin receptors. Transferrin is capable of binding two iron atoms per molecule and is reutilized after giving up iron to cells. The iron-responsive-element-binding protein (IRE-BP) is an RNA-binding protein which binds to specific messenger RNA sequences and is a mechanism whereby the body's iron content regulates uptake and storage of iron by cells of the RES. When iron is in excess, transferrin receptor synthesis, and therefore iron uptake, are reduced and ferritin synthesis is increased. Iron deficiency has the opposite effects.

Iron intake, absorption and loss

The average Western diet contains 10–15 mg of iron daily, of which 5–10% (about 1 mg) is normally absorbed through the upper small intestine. Absorption is adjusted to body needs (increased in iron deficiency and pregnancy, reduced in iron overload). Absorption is regulated by at least three proteins, DMT-1 at the villous tip and HFE and ferroportin 1 at the basolateral surfaces of the enterocyte. The DMT-1 level determines the amount of iron absorbed, and the DMT-1 level is in turn controlled by degree of expression of HFE. This is increased in iron deficiency. Iron in animal products is more easily absorbed than vegetable iron; inorganic iron in ferrous form is absorbed more than ferric form. Vitamin C enhances absorption; phytates inhibit it. Dietary intake makes up for daily loss (about 1 mg) in hair, skin, urine, faeces and menstrual blood loss in women. Infants, children and pregnant women need extra iron to expand their red cell mass and, in pregnancy, for transfer to the fetus.

Iron deficiency

Causes (Table 9.1)
- Blood loss (500 mL of normal blood contains 200–250 mg iron)—dominant cause in Western countries.
- Malabsorption—rarely a main cause.
- Poor dietary intake—a contributory cause, especially in

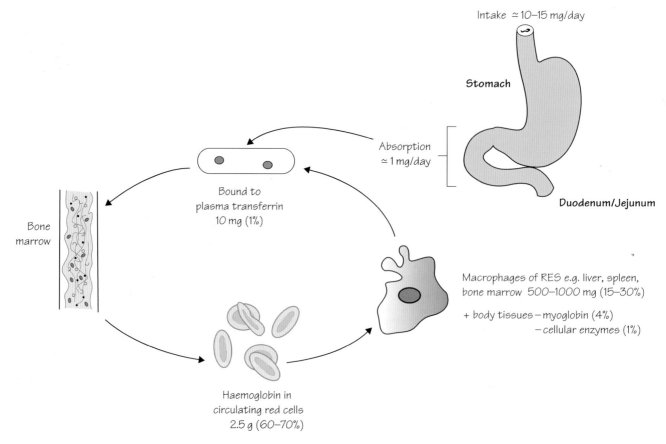

Fig. 9.1 Iron metabolism.

children, menstruating females or pregnancy, especially in developing countries.

Clinical features
- General features of anaemia (see Chapter 6).
- Special features (minority of patients): koilonychia (Fig. 9.2) or ridged brittle nails, glossitis, angular cheilosis (sore corners of mouth), pica (abnormal appetite), hair thinning and pharyngeal web formation (Paterson–Kelly syndrome).
- Features resulting from an underlying cause.

Laboratory findings
- Hypochromic microcytic anaemia.
- Raised platelet count.
- Blood film appearances (Fig. 9.3) include hypochromic/microcytic cells, aniso/poikilocytosis, target cells and 'pencil' cells.
- Bone marrow—not needed for diagnosis: erythroblasts show ragged irregular cytoplasm; absence of iron from stores and erythroblasts.
- Serum ferritin reduced, serum iron low with raised transferrin and unsaturated iron binding capacity.
- Serum soluble transferrin receptors increased.

Other investigations
- History (especially for blood loss, diet, malabsorption). Tests for cause (especially in males and postmenopausal females) include occult blood tests, upper and lower gastrointestinal endoscopy, tests for hookworm, malabsorption and for urine haemosiderin.

Table 9.1 Causes of iron deficiency.

Chronic blood loss

Uterine, e.g. menorrhagia or post-menopausal bleeding
Gastrointestinal, e.g. oesophageal varices, hiatus hernia, peptic ulcer, ingestion of aspirin (or other non-steroidal anti-inflammatory drugs), gastrectomy, carcinoma (stomach, caecum, colon or rectum), hookworm, angiodysplasia, colitis, diverticulosis, piles
Rarely, haematuria, haemoglobinuria, pulmonary haemosiderosis, self-inflicted blood loss

Increased demands

Prematurity ⎫
Growth ⎬ Deficiency occurs if these are associated with poor diet
Pregnancy ⎭

Malabsorption

Postgastrectomy, gluten-induced enteropathy

Poor diet

Rarely the sole cause in developed countries

- Haemoglobin electrophoresis and/or globin gene DNA analysis to exclude thalassaemia trait or other haemoglobin defects.

Treatment
- Oral iron—ferrous sulphate is best (200 mg, 67 mg iron per tablet) before meals three times daily.
- A reticulocyte response begins in 7 days but treatment should be continued for 4–6 months to replenish stores.
- Side effects (e.g. abdominal pain, diarrhoea or constipation) require a lower dose, taking iron with food, or a different preparation (e.g. ferrous gluconate 300 mg, 37 mg iron per tablet).
- Poor response may be due to continued bleeding, incorrect diagnosis, malabsorption or poor compliance.
- Prophylactic oral iron, often combined with folic acid, is given in pregnancy.
- Intramuscular iron is used in patients with malabsorption or who are unable to take oral iron. Intravenous iron may cause anaphylaxis but is useful to replenish iron stores in rare cases and in renal dialysis patients receiving erythropoietin therapy.

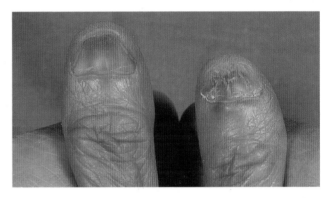

Fig. 9.2 Nail changes in chronic iron deficiency include brittle nails, ridged nails and spoon-shaped nails (koilonychia).

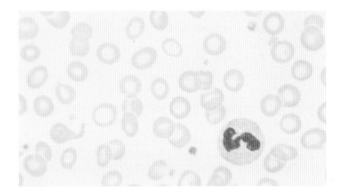

Fig. 9.3 Iron deficiency. Peripheral blood film showing hypochromic microcytic cells, with variation in cell size (anisocytosis) and abnormally shaped cells (poikilocytosis, e.g. pencil-shaped cells). Target cells are also seen in iron deficiency.

Iron overload

Iron overload is the pathological state in which total body stores of iron are increased, often with organ dysfunction as a result of iron deposition.

Causes

• Primary (genetic) haemochromatosis (GH) is an autosomal recessive condition associated with excessive iron absorption. Ninety percent of cases are homozygous for a mutation in the HFE gene situated close to the HLA complex on chromosome 6 (see Chapter 9).
• African iron overload; dietary and genetic components.
• Excess dietary iron.
• Ineffective erythropoiesis with increased iron absorption (e.g. thalassaemia intermedia).
• Repeated blood transfusions in patients with severe refractory anaemia, e.g. thalassaemia major, myelodysplasia. Each unit contains 250 mg iron.

Clinical features

• These are mainly caused by organ dysfunction as a result of iron deposition (Fig. 10.1).
• Cardiomyopathy gives rise to dysrhythmias and congestive heart failure: major cause of death.
• Growth/sexual development are reduced in children: delayed puberty, diabetes mellitus, hypothyroidism and hypoparathyroidism are frequent.
• The liver may show haemosiderosis and cirrhosis. The liver abnormality in transfusional iron overload is, however, often a result of hepatitis B or C infection.
• Excessive melanin skin pigmentation.
• Excessive infections.
• Arthropathy in GH caused by pyrophosphate deposition.

Laboratory features

• Raised serum iron and transferrin saturation.
• Raised serum ferritin.
• Lowered serum-soluble transferrin receptor level.
• Increased iron in liver and bone marrow (transfusional iron overload).
• Increased urinary iron excretion in response to iron chelator therapy.
• Abnormal liver function tests.
• Endocrine abnormalities, e.g. raised blood glucose.

Treatment

• Genetic haemochromatosis: regular venesections to reduce iron level to normal, assessed by serum ferritin, serum iron and total iron binding capacity and by liver biopsy.

• Transfusional iron overload: iron chelation using subcutaneous desferrioxamine (DFX) over 8–12 h on 5–7 nights each week. Vitamin C enhances iron excretion. An orally active iron chelator (deferiprone) is available for those unable to take DFX.

Sideroblastic anaemia

Definition

Sideroblastic anaemia is a refractory anaemia in which the marrow shows increased iron present as granules arranged in a ring around the nucleus in developing erythroblasts ('ringed sideroblasts', Fig. 10.2). At least 15% of erythroblasts show this in the primary forms. A defect of haem synthesis is present. Haem synthesis occurs in both the mitochondria and the cellular cytoplasm.

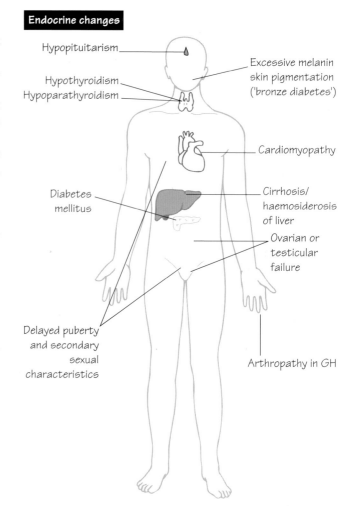

Endocrine changes

Hypopituitarism

Hypothyroidism
Hypoparathyroidism

Excessive melanin skin pigmentation ('bronze diabetes')

Cardiomyopathy

Diabetes mellitus

Cirrhosis/ haemosiderosis of liver

Ovarian or testicular failure

Delayed puberty and secondary sexual characteristics

Arthropathy in GH

Fig. 10.1 Iron overload: clinical features.

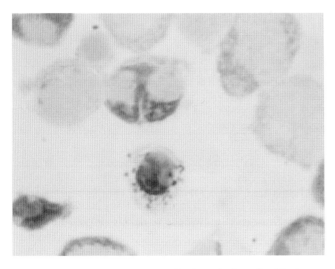

Fig. 10.2 Bone marrow iron stain (Perls' stain, Prussian blue) showing a ringed sideroblast.

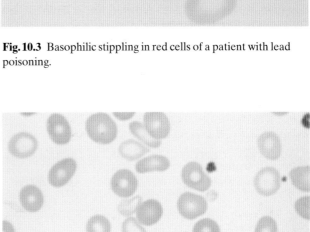

Fig. 10.3 Basophilic stippling in red cells of a patient with lead poisoning.

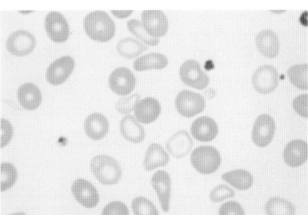

Fig. 10.4 Sideroblastic anaemia: dimorphic blood film. Dual population of well-haemoglobinized cells and hypochromic cells.

Classification
• The most common form is primary acquired type (a form of myelodysplasia; see Chapter 21).
• An X-linked genetic defect in haem synthesis (usually due to mutation of δ-amino laevulinic acid synthase, ALA-S), a key enzyme in haem synthesis underlies some congenital forms, usually in males.
• Ringed sideroblasts may also occur with other haematological disorders and with alcohol, isoniazid therapy and lead poisoning.

Clinical and laboratory features
The congenital anaemia is sometimes mild (haemoglobin 8–10 g/dL) but may become more severe with age. Leucopenia and thrombocytopenia may occur in patients with myelodysplasia. Blood film may be dimorphic (Fig. 10.4). The MCV is usually raised in acquired and low in the inherited variety.

Treatment
Usually symptomatic. Regular blood transfusion and iron chelation is often required. Patients with inherited forms may respond to pyridoxine (vitamin B_6), a co-factor for ALA-S.

Lead poisoning
Clinically this presents with abdominal pain, constipation, anaemia, peripheral neuropathy and a blue (lead) line of the gums. The blood film shows punctate basophilia (blue staining dots as a result of undegraded RNA) (Fig. 10.3) and features of haemolysis. The marrow may show ringed sideroblasts.

11 Megaloblastic anaemia I: Vitamin B$_{12}$ deficiency

Megaloblastic anaemia (MA) is associated with an abnormal appearance of the bone marrow erythroblasts in which nuclear development is delayed and nuclear chromatin has a lacy open appearance. There is a defect in DNA synthesis usually caused by deficiency of vitamin B$_{12}$ (B$_{12}$, cobalamin) or folate.

Biochemical basis

Folate is an essential coenzyme for the synthesis of thymidine monosphosphate (TMP) and therefore of DNA. B$_{12}$ is a coenzyme for methionine synthase, a reaction needed in the demethylation of the form of folate, 5-methyltetrahydrofolate (methyl THF), which enters the cells. The demethylation provides THF which acts as substrate for synthesis of intracellular folate polyglutamates, the coenzyme forms of folate needed in DNA synthesis.

B$_{12}$ physiology (Fig. 11.2)

• Adult daily requirement for B$_{12}$ is 1 μg (normal mixed diet contains 10–15 μg). B$_{12}$ is present only in foods of animal origin: meat, fish, eggs, milk and butter; it is absent from vegetables, cereals and fruit, unless contaminated by microorganisms. Normal body stores of B$_{12}$, largely in the liver with an enterohepatic circulation, are sufficient to last for 2–4 years.

• Dietary B$_{12}$ after release from food and gastric 'R' binder (see below) combines with intrinsic factor (IF) secreted by gastric parietal cells (GPC). IF–B$_{12}$ complex attaches to ileal receptors and B$_{12}$ is absorbed.

• Passive absorption (about 0.1% of oral B$_{12}$) occurs through buccal, gastric and duodenal mucosae.

• Absorbed B$_{12}$ attaches to transcobalamin (TC) II which carries B$_{12}$ in plasma to the liver, bone marrow, brain and other tissues. Most B$_{12}$ in plasma is attached to a second B$_{12}$ binding protein, TC I, and is functionally inactive. TC I is synthesized by granulocytes and their precursors. Similar glycoproteins ('R' proteins) occur in saliva, gastric juice and milk.

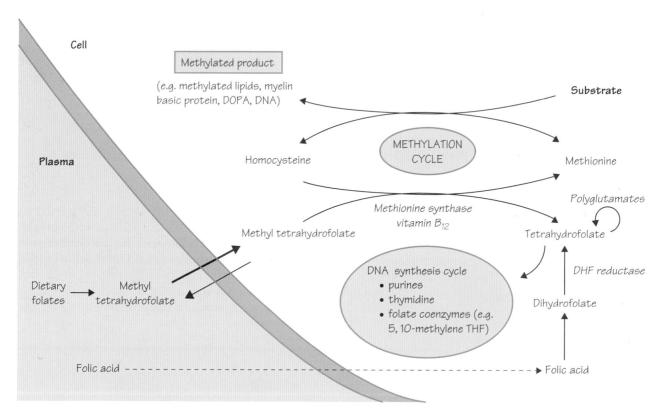

Fig. 11.1 The role of vitamin B$_{12}$ in conversion of 5-methyltetrahydrofolate to tetrahydrofolate required as substrate for folate polyglutamate synthesis. The reaction methionine synthase involves conversion of haemocysteine to methionine which is converted to *S*-adenosylmethionine involved in numerous methylation reactions. 5,10-Methylene tetrahydrofolate plays a key part in DNA synthesis by acting as coenzyme for synthesis of thymidine monophosphate from deoxyuridine monophosphate.

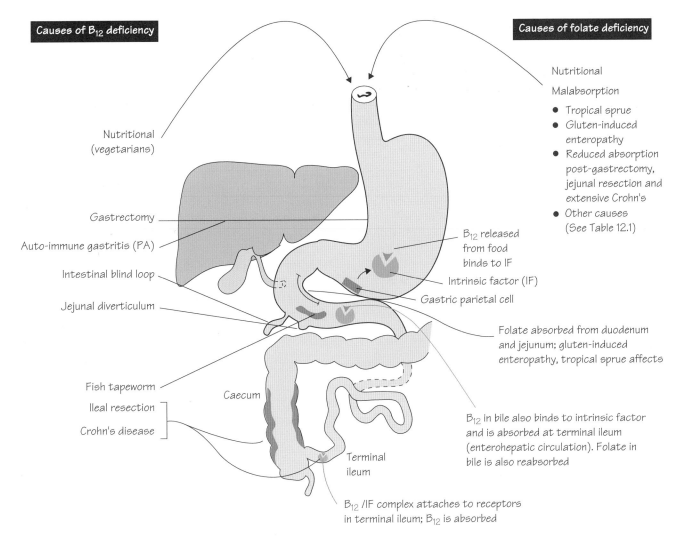

Causes of B₁₂ deficiency

Causes of B_{12} deficiency

Nutritional
(vegetarians)

Gastrectomy

Auto-immune gastritis (PA)

Intestinal blind loop

Jejunal diverticulum

Fish tapeworm

Ileal resection

Crohn's disease

Caecum

Terminal
ileum

Causes of folate deficiency

Nutritional

Malabsorption

- Tropical sprue
- Gluten-induced
  enteropathy
- Reduced absorption
  post-gastrectomy,
  jejunal resection and
  extensive Crohn's
- Other causes
  (See Table 12.1)

B_{12} released
from food
binds to IF

Intrinsic factor (IF)

Gastric parietal cell

Folate absorbed from duodenum
and jejunum; gluten-induced
enteropathy, tropical sprue affects

B_{12} in bile also binds to intrinsic factor
and is absorbed at terminal ileum
(enterohepatic circulation). Folate in
bile is also reabsorbed

B_{12}/IF complex attaches to receptors
in terminal ileum; B_{12} is absorbed

Fig. 11.2 The gastrointestinal tract in B_{12} or folate deficiency.

Causes of B_{12} deficiency

Inadequate diet

Vegans may develop B_{12} deficiency, although the intact enterohepatic circulation of a few microgrammes of B_{12} daily delays its onset. Infants born to B_{12}-deficient mothers and breast-fed by them may present with failure to thrive and MA resulting from B_{12} deficiency.

Malabsorption

Gastric causes

- Pernicious anaemia (PA) is characterized by an autoimmune gastritis, and reduced gastric secretion of IF and acid (Fig. 11.3). It is often associated with other organ-specific autoimmune diseases (e.g. myxoedema, thyrotoxicosis, vitiligo, Addison's disease and hypoparathyroidism). Antibodies to IF and gastric parietal cells occur in serum and in gastric secretion (50% and 90%, respectively) of patients. Pernicious anaemia is also associated with early greying of

hair, blue eyes, blood group A, a family history of PA or related autoimmune disease and a 2–3-fold increased incidence of carcinoma of the stomach. It occurs in all races and has a female/male incidence of 1.6:1. Peak age of incidence is 60 years.

- Gastrectomy (total or subtotal) leads to B_{12} deficiency.
- Congenital IF deficiency or abnormality is rare.

Intestinal causes

These include bacterial (rarely fish tapeworm) colonization of small intestine, stagnant loop syndromes, congenital and acquired defects of the ileum (e.g. ileal resection, Crohn's disease). Congenital B_{12} malabsorption with proteinuria is rare.

Clinical features

- Gradual onset of features of anaemia.
- Mild jaundice, caused by ineffective erythropoiesis.

- Glossitis (Fig. 11.3) and angular cheilosis and, if severe, sterility (either sex) and reversible melanin skin pigmentation.
- B$_{12}$ deficiency causes a symmetrical neuropathy affecting the pyramidal tracts and posterior columns of the spinal cord (subacute combined degeneration of the cord) and the peripheral nerves. Patients present with tingling in the feet (more than the hands), difficulty in gait, visual or psychiatric disorders.
- B$_{12}$ or folate deficiency are associated with increased plasma homocysteine which is associated with arterial and venous thrombosis and, in pregnancy, to an increased incidence of fetal neural tube defects.
- Patients may be asymptomatic and detected by a routine blood test.

Laboratory findings
- Macrocytic anaemia with oval macrocytes and hypersegmented neutrophils (>5 nuclear lobes) (Fig. 11.4).
- Moderate reduction in leucocyte and platelet counts (severe cases).
- Biochemical tests show raised serum bilirubin (indirect), lactate dehydrogenase.
- In B$_{12}$ deficiency, the serum B$_{12}$ is low, serum folate is normal or raised and red cell folate is normal or low.
- Bone marrow is hypercellular, increased proportion of early cells, megaloblastic erythropoiesis and giant metamyelocytes (Fig. 11.5).
- Raised serum methylmalonic acid (B$_{12}$ deficiency), raised serum homocysteine (either B$_{12}$ or folate deficiency).

Tests for causes of B$_{12}$ deficiency
These include history (diet, previous surgery), tests for IF and parietal cell antibodies, upper gastrointestinal endoscopy and radioactive B$_{12}$ absorption studies.

Radioactive B$_{12}$ absorption studies distinguish gastric

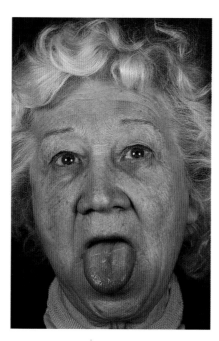

Fig. 11.3 Pernicious anaemia in a female aged 65 years. She is wearing a wig to disguise premature greying of the hair. There is a tinge of jaundice in the conjunctivae and skin, blue eyes and an enlarged fleshy sore tongue.

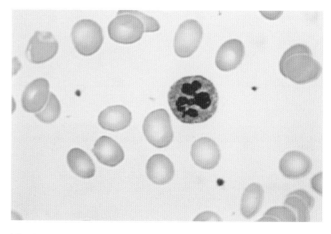

Fig. 11.4 Peripheral blood in megaloblastic anaemia, showing a hypersegmented neutrophil, oval macrocytes and poikilocytosis.

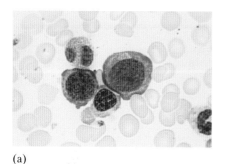

(a)

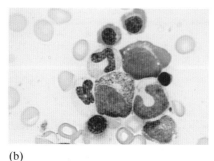

(b)

Fig. 11.5 (a) Bone marrow in megaloblastic anaemia showing megaloblasts. These are nucleated erythroid cells with open lacy chromatin and delayed nuclear maturation. (b) This shows megaloblasts with developing myeloid cells; the cell with a C-shaped nucleus is a giant metamyelocyte.

from intestinal causes of B_{12} malabsorption. The amount of radioactive B_{12} absorbed is measured either by whole body counting or in a 24-h urine sample after a 'flushing' dose of 1 mg unlabelled B_{12}, given simultaneously with the oral radioactive dose (Schilling test). The test can be performed with the labelled B_{12} given alone or with IF. A combined urinary excretion test using two isotopic forms of B_{12}, one bound to IF, can be used (Dicopac test). B_{12} absorption is low and corrected by IF in PA but is low and not corrected by IF in intestinal diseases.

Treatment

Treatment for B_{12} deficiency is 1 mg hydroxocobalamin intramuscularly, repeated every 2–3 days until six injections have been given; then one injection every 3 months for life unless the cause of deficiency has been corrected.

12 Megaloblastic anaemia II: Folate deficiency and other macrocytic anaemias

Physiology

Folates consist of a large number of compounds derived from the parent compound pteroylglutamic (folic) acid by reduction, addition of single carbon groups, e.g. methyl or formyl, and, in cells, addition of extra glutamate moieties usually four, five or six (see Fig. 11.1).
• Occur in most foods, especially liver and green vegetables. Normal daily diet contains 200–250 µg, of which about 50% is absorbed.
• Daily adult requirements are about 100 µg; body stores are sufficient for 4 months.
• Absorbed through the upper small intestine with conversion of all natural forms to 5-methyl tetrahydrofolate (methyl THF).

Clinical features

The clinical features of folate deficiency are the same as B_{12} deficiency, but folate deficiency does not cause a similar neuropathy. Folic acid therapy in early pregnancy reduces the incidence of neural tube defects (anencephaly, spina bifida, encephalocoele) in the fetus, probably by reducing homocysteine accumulation. Conversion of homocysteine to methionine requires the folate coenzyme methyl THF (see Fig. 11.1). Raised serum homocysteine is associated with vascular disease.

Causes of folate deficiency (Table 12.1)

• The most common cause is poor dietary intake, either alone or in association with increased folate utilization (e.g. pregnancy or haemolytic anaemia).
• Malabsorption occurs in gluten-induced enteropathy or tropical sprue.
• Increased utilization. Increased cell turnover and DNA synthesis causes breakdown of folates; the most common causes include pregnancy, haemolytic anaemia, severe chronic inflammatory and malignant diseases, and anticonvulsant drugs.
• Folate is loosely bound to protein in plasma and is easily removed by dialysis.

Tests for causes of deficiency

These include history (diet, previous surgery, drug therapy, alcohol, other associated diseases), antigliadin and endomysial antibodies, and tests for malabsorption (e.g. duodenal biopsy). The serum folate is low, red cell folate is low and serum B_{12} is normal or slightly reduced.

Treatment

Treatment is 5 mg folic acid daily for 4 months, then decide

Table 12.1 Causes of folate deficiency.

Nutritional

Especially old age, institutions, poverty, famine

Malabsorption

Gluten-induced enteropathy, dermatitis herpetiformis, tropical sprue

Excess utilization

Physiological
   Pregnancy and lactation, prematurity
Pathological
   Haematological diseases: haemolytic anaemias, myelofibrosis
   Malignant diseases: carcinoma, lymphoma, myeloma
   Inflammatory diseases: Crohn's disease, rheumatoid arthritis, extensive psoriasis, exfoliative dermatitis, malaria

Excess urinary folate loss

Congestive heart failure, chronic dialysis

Drugs

Anti-convulsants, sulphasalazine

Mixed

Liver disease, alcoholism (spirit drinkers)

whether to continue folic acid, e.g. 5 mg folic acid once weekly indefinitely. Folate therapy corrects the anaemia but not the neuropathy of B_{12} deficiency. Indeed, administration of folic acid to a severely B_{12}-deficient individual may precipitate or worsen B_{12} neuropathy. Pregnant women are given about 400 µg daily to reduce the incidence of megaloblastic anaemia and of neural tube defects in the fetus.

Other causes of megaloblastic anaemia

Defects of B_{12} or folate metabolism include congenital transcobalamin (TC) II deficiency which leads to B_{12} malabsorption and to failure of B_{12} to enter cells resulting in megaloblastic anaemia (MA) in early infancy. N_2O anaesthesia reversibly inactivates body B_{12} and prolonged or repeated exposure may cause megaloblastic anaemia or B_{12} neuropathy. Antifolate drugs include the inhibitors of dihydrofolate reductase (methotrexate, pyrimethamine and trimethoprim) which have progressively less activity against the human compared to the bacterial enzyme. Folinic acid (5-formyl-THF) is used to overcome methotrexate toxicity. Megaloblastic anaemia also occurs with cytotoxic drug therapy (e.g. 6-mercaptopurine, cytosine arabinoside or hydroxyurea (hydroxycarbamide)) or, rarely, inborn errors, e.g. orotic aciduria.

Causes of macrocytosis

Alcohol is the most frequent cause (Table 12.2). MCV is not usually as high as in severe MA in these conditions. White cell and platelet counts are normal unless the underlying marrow disease affects these, the red cells are circular rather than oval, hypersegmented neutrophils are absent and the marrow is normoblastic.

Table 12.2 Causes of raised MCV other than megaloblastic anaemia.

1 Alcohol
2 Liver disease
3 Myxoedema
4 Reticulocytosis
5 Cytoxic drugs
6 Aplastic anaemia
7 Pregnancy
8 Myelodysplastic syndromes
9 Myeloma
10 Neonatal

13 Haemolytic anaemias I: General

Haemolytic anaemias are caused by a shortened red cell lifespan; the normal mean red cell life (MRCL) is 120 days. Red cell production can be increased 6–8 times by normal bone marrow and haemolytic anaemia (HA) occurs if MRCL falls to 15 days or less, particularly in the presence of ineffective erythropoiesis, haematinic deficiency or marrow disease. Haemolysis may be caused by a fault in the red cell, usually inherited, or an abnormality in its environment, usually acquired (Table 13.1).

Physiology of red cell destruction (Fig. 13.1)

Red cell destruction is normally extravascular in the macrophages of the reticuloendothelial system, in bone marrow, liver and spleen. Globin is degraded to amino acids, haem to protoporphyrin, carbon monoxide and iron. Protoporphyrin is metabolized to bilirubin, conjugated to a glucuronide in the liver, excreted in faeces (as stercobilinogen) and, after reabsorption, in urine as urobilinogen. Iron is recycled to plasma and combined to transferrin. Some iron remains in the macrophages as ferritin and haemosiderin. Haptoglobins are plasma proteins which bind haemoglobin to form a complex which is removed by the liver; their level is reduced in haemolysis as well as in liver disease. Pathological red cell destruction may occur intravascularly (Table 13.2). Some haemoglobin is then excreted in the urine unchanged; it is also partly reabsorbed by the renal tubules and broken down to haemosiderin.

Table 13.1 Classification of haemolytic anaemia.

Hereditary	Acquired
Membrane	**Immune**
	Autoimmune
Hereditary spherocytosis, hereditary elliptocytosis	Warm antibody type Idiopathic or 2°-SLE, CLL, drugs e.g. methyldopa, fludarabine
South-East Asian ovalocytosis	Cold antibody type Idiopathic or 2°-infections (e.g. mycoplasma, infectious mononucleosis), lymphoma, paroxysmal cold haemoglobinuria
Metabolism	
G6PD deficiency	*Alloimmune*
Pyruvate kinase deficiency	Haemolytic transfusion reactions
Other rare enzyme deficiencies e.g. triose phosphate isomerase deficiency	Haemolytic disease of newborn
Haemoglobin	
Haemoglobin defect (HbS, HbC, unstable) see Chapter 17	**Red cell fragmentation syndromes**
	Cardiac valve, 'March' haemoglobinuria Thrombotic thrombocytopenia purpura Haemolytic uraemic syndrome Disseminated intravascular coagulation
	Infections
	e.g. malaria, clostridia
	Chemical and physical agents
	e.g. drugs, industrial/domestic substances, burns
	Secondary
	e.g. liver and renal disease
	Paroxysmal nocturnal haemoglobinuria (PNH)

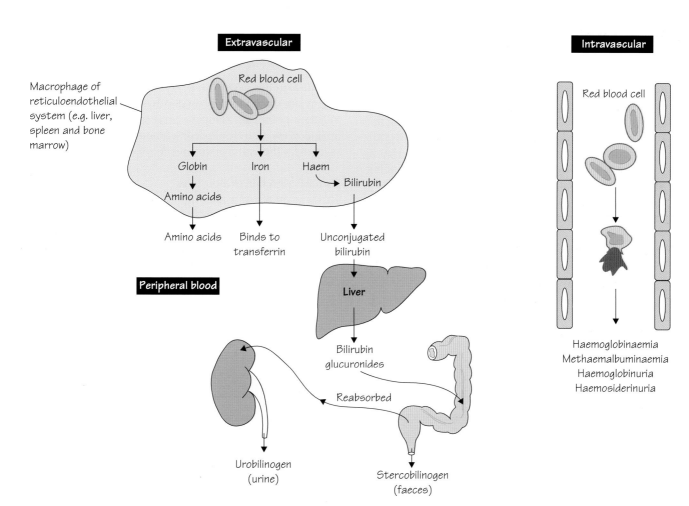

Fig. 13.1 Red cell breakdown.

Clinical features

- Anaemia (unless fully compensated haemolysis).
- Jaundice (usually mild) caused by unconjugated bilirubin in plasma; bilirubin is absent from the urine.
- An increased incidence of pigment gallstones.
- Splenomegaly — in many types.
- Ankle ulcers, especially sickle cell anaemia, thalassaemia intermedia and hereditary spherocytosis.
- Expansion of marrow with, in children, bone expansion e.g. frontal bossing in β thalassaemia major.
- Aplastic crises caused by parvovirus infection and megaloblastic anaemia caused by folate deficiency.

Laboratory features

- Haemoglobin level may be normal or reduced.
- Raised reticulocyte count.
- Blood film may show polychromasia (blue staining in young red cells), altered red cell shape, e.g. spherocytes, elliptocytes, sickle cells or fragmented cells.
- Bone marrow shows increased erythropoiesis.
- Serum indirect (unconjugated) bilirubin is raised.

Table 13.2 Causes of intravascular haemolysis.

Mismatched blood transfusion (usually ABO)
G6PD deficiency with oxidant stress
Red cell fragmentation syndromes
Some autoimmune haemolytic anaemias
Some drug- and infection-induced haemolytic anaemias
Paroxysmal nocturnal haemoglobinuria
March haemoglobinuria
Unstable haemoglobin

- Serum haptoglobins absent.
- Faecal stercobilinogen and urine urobilinogen are increased.
- Radioactive chromium (^{51}Cr) labelling of red cells measures lifespan and assesses the sites of red cell destruction by surface counting. Useful in predicting value of splenectomy.
- Intravascular haemolysis leads to raised plasma and urine haemoglobin, positive serum (Schumm's) test for methaemalbumin, urine haemosiderin.

14 Haemolytic anaemias II: Inherited membrane and enzyme defects

Membrane abnormalities

Hereditary spherocytosis (HS)

This is the most common inherited haemolytic anaemia (HA) in white people. It is autosomal dominant with variable severity and may present as severe neonatal HA, as symptomatic HA later in life, or as an incidental finding. Defect is in a red cell membrane protein e.g. ankyrin; 25% of cases are new mutations. Affected red cells lose membrane during passage through the reticuloendothelial system, especially the spleen. The cells become progressively more spherical (decreased surface area/volume ratio) and microcytic. They are destroyed prematurely, mainly in the spleen.

Clinical features

Clinical features are those generally associated with HA. The spleen is usually enlarged.

Laboratory features

- Blood film: microspherocytes and polychromasia (Fig. 14.1).
- Haemoglobin level variable.
- Tests for HA are positive (see Chapter 13).
- Special tests: osmotic fragility increased (Fig. 14.2), autohaemolysis increased and corrected by addition of glucose.
- Direct antiglobulin test is negative (excluding warm autoimmune HA which can cause a similar blood picture).

Treatment

- Splenectomy corrects the decrease in lifespan although spherocytosis persists; may not be needed in mild cases; defer if possible in children until over the age of 6 years.
- Give folic acid prophylactically for severe cases.
- Pigment gallstones may cause cholecystitis.
- If cholecystectomy required, perform splenectomy also to reduce risk of recurrent gallstones.

Hereditary elliptocytosis (HE) (Fig. 14.3)

This is similar but usually milder than HS. It is usually due to a spectrin defect. The peripheral blood is characteristic. Splenectomy is rarely needed. A homozygous form causes a severe HA (hereditary pyropoikilocytosis).

South-East Asian ovalocytosis

This is an inherited red cell membrane protein defect (band 3), in which carriers have a degree of protection against malaria.

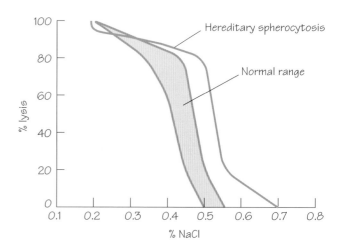

Fig. 14.2 Osmotic fragility test. Red cells are suspended in saline of increasing concentration and the degree of haemolysis is assessed by spectrophotometry. The red cells of patients with hereditary spherocytosis have an increased volume/surface area ratio and are more susceptible to lysis than normal red blood cells.

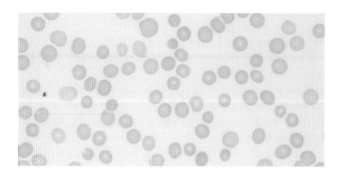

Fig. 14.1 Hereditary spherocytosis: peripheral blood film.

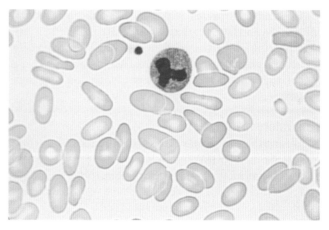

Fig. 14.3 Hereditary elliptocytosis: peripheral blood film.

Enzyme abnormalities

Glucose-6-phosphate dehydrogenase (G6PD) deficiency

G6PD is the first enzyme in the hexose monophosphate pathway (see Fig. 2.4) which generates reducing power as reduced nicotinamide adenine dinucleotide phosphate (NADPH). Deficiency results in red cells being susceptible to oxidant stress. The gene is on the X chromosome so inheritance is sex-linked. Many mutant enzymes occur. Affected males develop HA when the red cells are exposed to oxidant stress, especially by drugs, infections, ingestion of fava beans and during the neonatal period (Table 14.1). Deficiency is common in black, mediterranean, middle-eastern and oriental populations. There is epidemiological evidence that individuals with G6PD deficiency have a degree of protection against malaria.

Clinical and laboratory features
- Blood count and film normal between crises.
- During crises features of acute intravascular haemolysis.
- Blood film in a crisis (see Fig. 14.4) shows red cells with absent haemoglobin ('bite' and 'blister' cells) and polychromasia. Heinz bodies (denatured haemoglobin) may be seen in a reticulocyte preparation with supravital staining.
- Haemolysis is usually self-limited because of the increased G6PD activity in reticulocytes.
- Chronic non-spherocytic HA (CNSHA) occurs rarely with certain mutant enzymes.
- Neonatal jaundice is frequent.
- Screening tests for red cell G6PD deficiency measure the generation of NADPH. The enzyme may also be characterized by electrophoresis, assay of activity and DNA analysis. Diagnosis should, when possible, be undertaken in the steady state as reticulocytes generally have higher enzyme activity and the raised reticulocyte count following haemolysis may lead to a false normal result.

Management
- Stop offending drugs or fava bean ingestion.
- Treat infection if present.
- Transfuse packed red cells if necessary.
- Splenectomy may ameliorate HA in rare CNSHA.

Pyruvate kinase deficiency

Pyruvate kinase (PK) deficiency is the most frequent enzyme deficiency in the Embden–Meyerhof (glycolytic) pathway to cause CNSHA (see Fig. 14.5). Inheritance is autosomal recessive. The O_2-dissociation curve is shifted to the right so symptoms are mild in comparison to the degree of anaemia. Splenectomy partly improves the anaemia.

Other enzyme deficiencies are rare causes of CNSHA and are frequently associated with musculoskeletal disease.

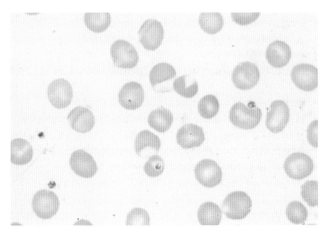

Fig. 14.4 Glucose-6-phosphate dehydrogenase deficiency: peripheral blood film showing red cells which have 'blistered' cytoplasm, and where haemoglobin in cytoplasm is contracted and pulled away from the membrane to give a 'basket' cell.

Table 14.1 Agents which may cause haemolytic anaemia in G6PD deficiency.

Infections and other acute illnesses, e.g. diabetic ketoacidosis
Drugs
    Antimalarials, e.g. primaquine
    Sulphonamides and sulphones, e.g. cotrimoxazole,
        sulphanilamide, dapsone, salazopyrine
    Other antibacterial agents, e.g. nitrofurans, chloramphenicol
    Analgesics, e.g. aspirin (moderate doses are safe)
    Antihelminths, e.g. β-naphthol, stibophen, niridazole
    Miscellaneous, e.g. vitamin K analogues, naphthalene
        (mothballs), probenecid
Fava beans (possibly other vegetables)

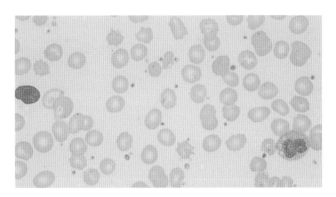

Fig. 14.5 Pyruvate kinase deficiency: peripheral blood film, postsplenectomy, showing irregularly contracted and crenated 'spicule' cells or 'prickle' cells—an extreme type of ecchinocyte.

15 Haemolytic anaemias III: Acquired

Autoimmune haemolytic anaemia

This is caused by autoantibodies against the red cell membrane. It is divided into warm and cold antibody types and each may be idiopathic or secondary to other diseases (see Table 13.1).

Warm autoimmune haemolytic anaemia

Antibody, typically IgG, has maximum activity at 37°C.

Clinical and laboratory features
- Presents at any age, in either sex, with features of extravascular haemolytic anaemia of varying severity.
- The spleen is often enlarged.
- Blood film shows microspherocytes (Fig. 15.1), polychromasia, anisocytosis, ±circulating nucleated red blood cells.
- Direct antiglobulin test (DAT) is positive (Fig. 15.2).
- Antibody may be non-specific or directed against antigens in the Rh system.
- IgG or IgG + complement (C3d) is detected on the red cell.
- Free antibody may be present in the serum.
- May be associated with immune thrombocytopenia (Evans' syndrome).
- Antibody-coated red cells are destroyed in the reticuloendothelial system, especially the spleen.

Treatment
- Corticosteroids, e.g. prednisolone 1 mg/kg orally with subsequent gradual reduction.
- Blood transfusion if necessary.
- Consider splenectomy if steroid therapy fails.
- Other immunosuppressive drugs, e.g. azathioprine, cyclosporin, cyclophosphamide.

- Remove cause, e.g. drug.
- Treat underlying disease, e.g. chronic lymphocytic leukaemia (CLL), systemic lupus erythematosus.

Cold autoimmune haemolytic anaemia

Antibody, typically IgM, has maximum activity at 4°C.

Clinical and laboratory features (Fig. 15.3)
- Raynaud's phenomenon affecting the fingers, toes, nose and ears.
- Positive DAT with C3d on red cells.
- Cold agglutinins, usually IgM and directed against I or i antigen (especially in infectious mononucleosis) on red

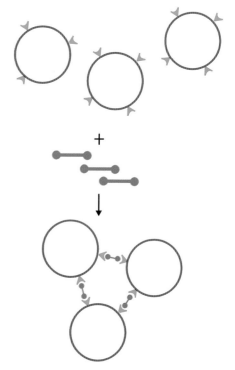

↬ Anti-human globulin (AHG, Coombs' reagent)

◄ Antibody (IgG, IgM or IgA) or complement coating RBC

○ Red blood cell

Fig. 15.2 Direct antiglobulin (Coombs') test (DAT) is a means of detecting immunoglobulin and/or complement coating the red blood cells. Red blood cells are washed and anti-human globulin is added. This may be of broad specificity or specific, e.g. for IgG, IgA, IgM or complement. If agglutination occurs, then the red blood cells must have been coated; if no agglutination occurs, the red blood cells were not coated. In the indirect antiglobulin test, red cells are first incubated with serum at 37°C for 30 min; a DAT is then performed, which will be positive if there are antibodies in the serum reacting against the red blood cells.

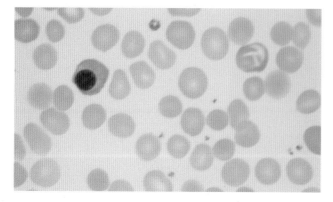

Fig. 15.1 Warm autoimmune haemolytic anaemia: peripheral blood film. There is a circulating nucleated red blood cell (NRBC), polychromasia and microspherocytes.

cells are present in serum, often to titres of 1:4000 or more. In primary form (cold haemagglutinin disease) the antibody is monoclonal and the patient may ultimately develop non-Hodgkin lymphoma.

• Paroxysmal cold haemoglobinuria is a rare syndrome, precipitated by infections. Intravascular haemolysis is caused by the Donath–Landsteiner antibody which binds red cells in the cold but causes lysis at 37°C.

Treatment
• Keep the patient warm.
• Consider immunosuppression with chlorambucil or cyclophosphamide.
• Consider plasma exchange to lower antibody titre.

Alloimmune haemolytic anaemia

This is caused when antibody produced by one individual reacts against red cells of another. The three important situations are:
1 mismatched blood transfusions (see Chapter 37);
2 haemolytic disease of the newborn (see Chapter 37); and
3 following marrow or solid organ transplantation.

Drug-induced immune haemolytic anaemia

Mechanisms include the following.
• Antibody directed against a drug (e.g. penicillin)–red cell membrane complex, the drug acting as a hapten.
• Antibody against a drug (e.g. quinidine)–plasma protein complex with subsequent deposition of the immune complex on red cells.
• Stimulation of autoantibody (warm type) production against the red cell, e.g. methyldopa, fludarabine.

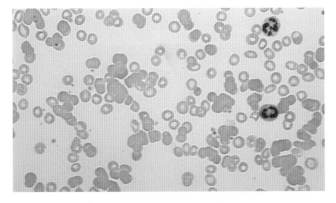

Fig. 15.3 Cold agglutinins: peripheral blood film. This patient developed anaemia 7 days after recovering from mycoplasma pneumonia; investigations revealed a cold autoantibody of anti-I specificity which was causing a low-grade haemolytic anaemia. Red cell agglutinates disappear if a blood film is prepared at 37°C.

Red cell fragmentation syndromes

These occur when red cells are exposed to an abnormal surface (e.g. non-endothelialized artificial heart valve or arterial graft), or flow through small vessels containing fibrin strands (e.g. in disseminated intravascular coagulation) or damaged small vessels. This is termed microangiopathic haemolytic anaemia (MAHA) and occurs in thrombotic thrombocytopenic purpura, haemolytic uraemic syndrome, widespread adenocarcinoma, malignant hypertension, pre-eclampsia and meningococcal septicaemia. Haemolysis is both extra- and intravascular; blood film shows deeply staining fragmented red cells (see Fig. 29.5).

Infections

These may cause haemolysis by:
• direct damage to red cells (e.g. malaria);
• toxin production (e.g. clostridium perfringens);
• oxidant stress in G6PD-deficient individuals;
• MAHA (e.g. meningococcal septicaemia);
• autoantibody formation (e.g. infectious mononucleosis);
• extravascular destruction (e.g. malaria).

Chemical and physical agents

Some drugs, e.g. dapsone, or chemicals, e.g. chlorate, cause haemolysis by oxidation even with normal G6PD levels. Severe burns and snake bites may also cause haemolysis.

Paroxysmal nocturnal haemoglobinuria

This is a clonal disorder in which haemolysis is caused by a rare acquired mutation of the PIG-A gene in haemopoietic stem cells. This results in a defect of the phosphatidyl inositol anchor which tethers a large number of proteins to the cell membrane. The cells become abnormally sensitive to complement-mediated haemolysis (lack of proteins that protect against complement, e.g. MIRL, DAF). It is often associated with a hypoplastic marrow with neutropenia and thrombocytopenia. The clinical course is frequently complicated by recurrent venous thromboses, especially of large veins, e.g. hepatic or portal; also by iron deficiency and infections. Diagnosis is made by a positive acid lysis (Ham's) test and the presence of red cells lacking the MIRL or DAF antigens.

Treatment
• Iron is given for iron deficiency resulting from chronic intravascular haemolysis.
• Transfusion of leucodepleted red cells may be necessary.
• Warfarin may be needed life-long to prevent thrombosis.
• Allogeneic stem cell transplant for serious cases in young adults.

Genetic disorders of haemoglobin comprise:

1 disorders of globin chain synthesis (the thalassaemias);
2 structural defects of haemoglobin which give rise to haemolysis (e.g. sickle cell anaemia, haemoglobin C);
3 unstable haemoglobins (rare); and
4 structural disorders giving rise to polycythaemia or methaemoglobinaemia (rare).

The first and second have a wide global prevalence, particularly where malaria is, or was, common, as the carrier states give some protection against falciparum malaria. Frequent compound heterozygotes of a thalassaemic allele and a haemoglobin structural variant allele include sickle/β-thalassaemia and Hb E/β-thalassaemia.

Thalassaemia

These autosomal recessive syndromes divide into α- and β-thalassaemia depending on whether there is reduced synthesis of α- or β-globin (Table 16.1).

α-thalassaemia

Normally there are four α-globin genes, two on each chromosome 16 (see Fig. 2.2). Severity of α-thalassaemia depends on the number of α-genes deleted or, less frequently, dysfunctional.

Hydrops fetalis

In hydrops fetalis all four α genes are inactive. The fetus is unable to make either fetal ($\alpha_2 \gamma_2$) or adult Hb A ($\alpha_2 \beta_2$) haemoglobin. Death occurs *in utero* or neonatally.

Haemoglobin H disease

This is caused by deletion or functional inactivity of three of the four α genes. Markedly microcytic hypochromic anaemia (Hb 6–11.0 g/dL); splenomegaly usual. Bone deformities and features of iron overload do not occur. Haemoglobin electrophoresis shows 4–10% haemoglobin H (β_4) and supravital staining shows 'golf ball' cells.

α-thalassaemia trait

This is a one or two α gene deletion with microscopic hypochromic red cells with raised red cell count ($>5.5 \times 10^9$/L). Mild anaemia occurs in some cases with two α genes deleted.

β-thalassaemia

Thalassaemia major

Complete (βo) or almost complete (β+) failure of β-globin chain synthesis resulting from one of nearly 200 different point mutations or deletions in the β-globin gene or its controlling sequences on chromosome 11. There is severe imbalance of $\alpha : \beta + \gamma$ chains with deposition of α chains in erythroblasts, ineffective erythropoiesis, severe anaemia and extramedullary haemopoiesis.

Clinical features

• Anaemia presents at the age of 3–6 months when the switch from γ- to β-chain synthesis normally occurs. Milder cases present later (up to age 4 years).
• Failure to thrive, intercurrent infection, pallor, mild jaundice.
• Enlargement of the liver and spleen, expansion of the bones—especially of the skull—with bossing and a 'hair on

Table 16.1 Classification of thalassaemia.

Clinical phenotype	Thalassaemia (thal) syndrome
Hydrops fetalis	Homozygous α-thal major → complete lack of α globin
Thalassaemia major	Homozygous β or doubly heterozygous thal major → complete or almost complete lack of β globin
Thalassaemia intermedia	See p. 49
Thalassaemia trait	Heterozygous β-thalassaemia (β-thal minor, lack of one functional β-globin gene*)
	Heterozygous α-thalassaemia (α-thal minor, lack of one or two α-globin genes†)

* Normal individual has two (one from each parent/on each allele).

† Normal individual has four (two from each parent on each allele).

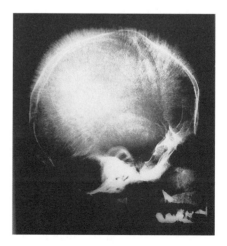

Fig. 16.1 β-thalassaemia major: skull X-ray showing expansion of the medullary cavity giving rise to a 'hair on end' appearance.

end' appearance on X-ray (Fig. 16.1); thalassaemic facies, caused by expansion of skull and facial bones.
• Features of iron overload as a result of blood transfusions include melanin pigmentation, growth/endocrine defects, cardiac failure, liver abnormality (see Chapter 10).

Laboratory findings
• Severe anaemia (Hb 2–6 g/dL) with reduced MCV and MCH.
• Blood film (Fig. 16.2) shows hypochromic microcytic cells, target cells, erythroblasts and, often, myelocytes.
• Bone marrow is hypercellular with erythroid hyperplasia.
• Globin chain synthesis studies show absent, or severely deficient, β-chain synthesis. Fetal haemoglobin variably increased.
• DNA analysis reveals the specific mutations or deletions.

Management
• Regular transfusions of packed red cells to maintain haemoglobin above 9–10 g/dL, leucodepleted to reduce risk of HLA sensitization and of transmission of disease, e.g. cytomegalovirus.
• Iron chelation therapy with subcutaneous desferrioxamine (DFX) over 8–12 h on 5–7 nights weekly. Additional DFX may be given intravenously at the time of blood transfusion via a separate bag. Oral vitamin C increases iron excretion with DFX. An orally active chelator, deferiprone is also available for those unable to take DFX (see also Chapter 10).
• Hepatitis B is prevented by early immunization. Patients who already have chronic active hepatitis caused by hepatitis C may need α-interferon + ribavirin therapy.
• Splenectomy is necessary if blood requirements are excessively high. Defer if possible until the age of 5 years, precede by immunization (see Chapter 39) and follow by oral penicillin therapy for life. If the platelet count remains raised, low-dose aspirin reduces the risk of thromboembolism.
• Bone marrow transplantation from an HLA-matching sibling may give long-term disease-free survival of up to 90% in good-risk patients, but nearer 50% in poor risk (previously poorly chelated with enlarged liver and liver fibrosis).
• Treat complications of iron overload: heart, endocrine organs, liver damage.
• Osteoporosis may occur as a result of marrow expansion, endocrine deficiencies.

Thalassaemia intermedia
A variable syndrome milder than thalassaemia major, with later onset, and characterized by moderately severe (Hb

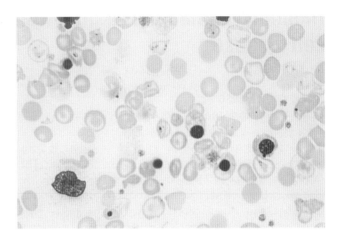

Fig. 16.2 β-thalassaemia major: peripheral blood film showing hypochromic microcytic red cells, target cells, poikilocytes and nucleated red blood cells. The few well-haemoglobinized cells are transfused red cells.

6–10 g/dL), hypochromic microcytic anaemia requiring either few or no transfusions. There is milder imbalance of α:β+γ globin chain synthesis than in thalassaemia major due to milder β-chain defects, increased γ chains or reduced α-chain synthesis. Hepatosplenomegaly, extramedullary haemopoiesis, anaemia and bone deformities may occur. Iron overload occurs as a result of irregular blood transfusions and increased gastrointestinal iron absorption.

β-thalassaemia trait
A mild hypochromic microcytic anaemia with a raised red cell count ($>5.5 \times 10^{12}$/L) and raised haemoglobin A_2 ($\alpha_2 \delta_2$) level ($>3.5\%$). Iron stores are normal, though iron deficiency may occur as in unaffected subjects. Accurate diagnosis allows genetic counselling and avoidance of inappropriate iron therapy.

Prenatal diagnosis of haemoglobin defects
Prenatal diagnosis is available using either DNA (chorionic villous or amniotic fluid) or fetal blood. Carriers must first be identified (screening by blood count in ethnic minority groups, at preconception counselling or in the antenatal clinic). If a mother is a carrier, her partner must be tested. If both are carriers, there is a one in four chance that the fetus is homozygous, or doubly heterozygous, and a one in two chance that the fetus is a carrier. Fetal DNA is then usually amplified by use of the polymerase chain reaction and the DNA mutations are detected. If the fetus is severely affected the couple should be counselled and termination of pregnancy, if appropriate, offered.

17 Haemolytic anaemias V: Inherited defects of haemoglobin—sickle cell disease

Sickle cell disease

Sickle cell disease (homozygous sickle cell anaemia) is a chronic haemolytic anaemia caused by a point mutation in the β-globin gene causing substitution of valine for glutamic acid in the sixth position of the β-globin chain. This causes insolubility of Hb S in its deoxygenated state. The insoluble chains crystallize in the red cells causing sickling (Fig. 17.1) and vascular occlusion. The disease is most common in Africans (1 in 5 West Africans are carriers—they have some protection against falciparum malaria). The mutant gene also occurs in other parts of the world where malaria is or was prevalent, e.g. the Middle East, Far East and the Indian subcontinent.

Clinical features

These resemble those of other chronic haemolytic anaemias, punctuated with different types of crisis.

1 Vaso-occlusive with blockage of small vessels is caused by increased sickling; common precipitants are infection, dehydration, acidosis and deoxygenation. Abdominal pain is caused by infarction affecting abdominal organs; bone pain may occur in the back, pelvis, ribs and long bones. Infarction may affect the central nervous system—causing a stroke or fits—lungs, spleen or kidneys. In children the 'hand–foot syndrome' is caused by infarction of the metaphyses of the small bones.

2 Visceral sequestration crisis is caused by sickling with pooling of red cells in the liver, spleen or lungs. Sequestration in the lungs is partly responsible for the acute chest syndrome, though infarction and infection contribute.

3 Aplastic crisis occurs following infection by B19 parvovirus. This causes temporary arrest of erythropoiesis which in healthy individuals is of no consequence but in patients with reduced red cell survival, such as Hb SS, can rapidly cause severe anaemia requiring blood transfusion.

• Increased susceptibility to infection. Splenic function is reduced because infarction leads to autosplenectomy in severe cases in infancy. Pneumococcal infections may lead to pneumonia and meningitis. Infarction of intestinal mucosa predisposes to *Salmonella* infection and osteomyelitis may result.

• Other clinical features include pigment gallstones with cholecystitis, chronic leg ulcers, avascular necrosis of the femoral and humeral heads (Fig. 17.2) or other bones, cardiomyopathy, proliferative retinopathy and renal papillary necrosis (leading to polyuria, failure to concentrate urine and tendency to dehydration).

Laboratory features

• Haemoglobin level is 7–9 g/dL but symptoms of anaemia are usually mild (the O_2 dissociation curve of Hb S is shifted to the right).

• Blood film shows sickle cells, target cells and often features of splenic atrophy (see Fig. 17.1).

• Screening tests for sickling demonstrate increased turbidity of the blood after deoxygenation (e.g. with dithionate or Na_2HPO_4). Haemoglobin electrophoresis (Fig. 17.5) shows haemoglobin with an abnormal migration. In Hb SS there is absence of Hb A. Hb F level is usually mildly raised (5–10%).

Treatment

• General—avoid known precipitants of sickle cell crisis,

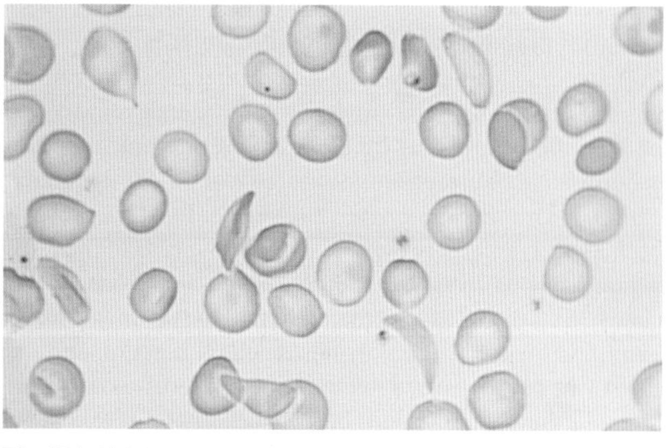

Fig. 17.1 Sickle cell anaemia (Hb SS): peripheral blood film showing sickle cells, anisocytois and changes of hyposplenism (target cells, Howell–Jolly bodies).

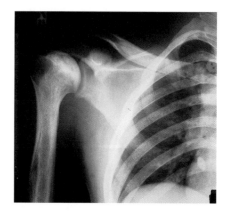

Fig. 17.2 Sickle cell anaemia: bony changes. X-ray showing avascular necrosis of the head of the humerus.

especially dehydration and infections. Give folic acid, pneumococcal, HIB and meningococcal vaccination and oral penicillin indefinitely to compensate for splenic atrophy.

• Vaso-occlusive crisis is treated with hydration, usually intravenous normal saline, analgesia (e.g. diamorphine subcutaneous infusion); O_2 if there is hypoxia; antibiotics if there is infection.

• Red cell transfusion for severe anaemia (sequestration or aplastic crisis) or as a 3–6-month programme of therapy for patients with frequently recurring crises or for 2–3 years following central nervous system crisis.

• Severe sickling or sequestration crisis (e.g. 'chest syndrome' and stroke) is treated acutely with exchange transfusion to reduce Hb S levels to <30%. Pregnant patients and those undergoing general anaesthesia may need transfusion to reduce Hb S levels to <30%.

• Oral hydroxyurea (20–40 mg/kg/day) reduces both the frequency and duration of sickle cell crisis. Although its precise mode of action is not known, it increases Hb F production, decreases intracellular Hb S concentration by increasing MCV, lowers the neutrophil count and inhibits prothrombotic interactions between sickle cells and the endothelium.

• Bone marrow transplantation in selected cases.

• Joint replacement surgery may be required for avascular necrosis (hips and shoulder).

• Iron chelation therapy for patients with iron overload caused by multiple transfusions.

Sickle cell trait

Sickle cell trait is a benign condition without anaemia and is usually asymptomatic. Occasionally haematuria or overt crisis occurs. Genetic counselling should be offered to carriers.

Other sickling disorders

Haemoglobin S may occur in combination with other genetic defects of haemoglobin (compound heterozygotes). Hb S/β-thalassaemia (Fig. 17.3) clinically resembles Hb SS but the spleen usually remains enlarged and MCV is reduced. Hb SC (Fig. 17.4) disease varies in severity from mild to indistinguishable from sickle cell anaemia; thrombotic complications are particularly common.

Other structural haemoglobin abnormalities

Many other mutations of the α- or β-chain genes have been identified. Most that have a significant population frequency are not associated with clinical symptoms.

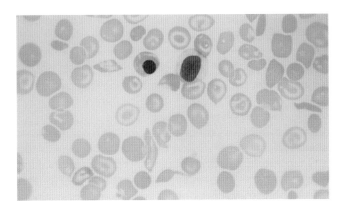

Fig. 17.3 Sickle cell/β-thalassaemia (Hb S/β-thal): peripheral blood film. Target cells, hypochromasia and a low mean corpuscular volume (MCV) are characteristic.

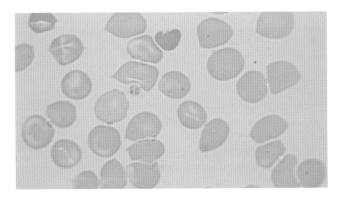

Fig. 17.4 Sickle cell/haemoglobin C (Hb SC): peripheral blood film showing fewer sickle cells densely staining irregularly contracted cells, boat-shaped cells, fewer hyposplenic changes and fewer nucleated red blood cells.

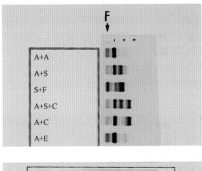
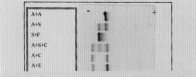

Fig. 17.5 Haemoglobin electrophoresis (Hb Ep). A lysate of red cells is applied to a gel and an electronic current is applied. The upper panel shows migration of different haemoglobins in acid agar gel (pH 6.0) and the lower panel shows migration in cellulose acetate at alkaline pH. Haemoglobins S and D and haemoglobins A_2, C and E run together on cellulose acetate and must be distinguished by acid agar Hb Ep.

18 Bone marrow failure

Bone marrow failure is the failure of the bone marrow to produce sufficient red cells, white cells and platelets. Causes are listed in Table 18.1. The bone marrow may be hypoplastic or aplastic, with a reduction in haemopoietic cells and an increase in fat spaces. Alternatively, the haemopoietic cells may be replaced by abnormal cells or malignant cells either arising in the marrow (primary) or infiltrating it (secondary).

Clinical features
• Symptoms and signs of anaemia, infections and easy bruising or bleeding.
• Symptoms and signs as a result of the underlying cause, e.g. side effects of chemotherapy.

Laboratory findings
• Anaemia, leucopenia and thrombocytopenia of varying severity.
• Blood film may show circulating red cell and white precursors (leucoerythroblastic) caused by bone marrow infiltration (see Chapter 34) or may show evidence of primary haematological malignancy, e.g. circulating leukaemic blast cells.
• Bone marrow aspirate and trephine biopsy are required to define cause (Fig. 18.1).

Differential diagnosis
• Pancytopenia (reduction in all three haemopoietic cell lines) can also result from accelerated destruction of cells (e.g. as a result of splenomegaly or autoimmune destruction) or pooling of cells (e.g. within an enlarged spleen).

Treatment
• Remove any known cause, e.g. drugs.

Table 18.1 Bone marrow failure.

Primary reduction in haemopoietic cells

Aplastic anaemia

Replacement of marrow by malignant cells

Primary—leukaemia, myeloma, lymphoma
Secondary—e.g. carcinoma

Ineffective haemopoiesis

Myelodysplasia, megaloblastic anaemia

Infiltration by abnormal tissue

Myelofibrosis
Rarely, Gaucher's disease, amyloidosis, osteopetrosis

• Support care with appropriate blood components (see Chapter 37) and antimicrobials (see Chapter 39).
• Specific therapy is considered separately with the specific diseases.

Aplastic anaemia
This is a chronic pancytopenia associated with a hypoplastic bone marrow. There are reduced marrow stem cells, increased fat spaces (fat/haemopoiesis ratio >75:25%) and no evidence of malignancy. The marrow microenvironment is intact.

Aetiology and pathogenesis
The disease may be congenital or acquired (Table 18.2).
• Congenital aplastic anaemia may be inherited as an autosomal recessive (Fanconi type); rarely associated with dyskeratosis congenita.
• Acquired aplastic anaemia has an identifiable cause (viral infection, radiation or drug exposure) in about 50% of cases. In the remainder the cause is unknown, but may involve an immune reaction against marrow stem cells.

Clinical features
• May occur at any age, in either sex, incidence of 2–5 cases/million population.
• Onset rapid (over a few days) or slow (over weeks or months).
• Symptoms and signs are caused by bone marrow failure (see above).
• Liver, spleen and lymph nodes are not enlarged.

Table 18.2 Causes of aplastic anaemia.

Congenital

Fanconi
Other, e.g. dyskeratosis congenita

Acquired

Idiopathic
Secondary
  Inevitable (cytotoxic drugs, radiation)
  Idiosyncratic
    Drugs, e.g. chlorampenicol, sulphonamides, gold, chlorpromazine, carbimazole
    Chemical agents/toxins, e.g. benzene
    Infection, e.g. viral hepatitis (non-A, non-B, non-C)
Associated with haematological malignancy, e.g. acute lymphoblastic leukaemia
Other, e.g. in association with paroxysmal nocturnal haemoglobinuria

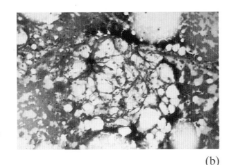

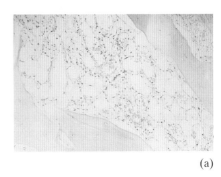

Fig. 18.1 Aplastic anaemia: (a) bone marrow aspirate; and (b) trephine biopsy showing reduced cellularity with increased fat spaces.

(b)

(a)

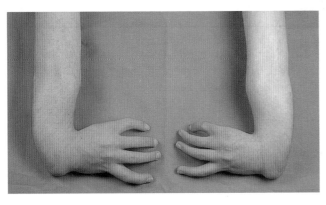

Fig. 18.2 Aplastic anaemia: Fanconi's anaemia, with multiple skeletal deformities of upper limbs.

• Fanconi's anaemia (Fig. 18.2) usually presents in childhood. Associated findings may include skeletal and renal tract defects, microcephaly and altered skin pigmentation. In dyskeratosis congenita there are skin, hair and nail changes.

Laboratory findings
• Anaemia is normocytic or mildly macrocytic with a low reticulocyte count.
• Leucopenia is usual with neutrophils below 1.5×10^9/L ($<0.2 \times 10^9$/L in severe cases).
• Thrombocytopenia ($<10 \times 10^9$/L in severe cases).
• Bone marrow is hypoplastic with >75% fat spaces. Remaining haemopoietic cells are of normal appearance. Megakaryocytes are particularly reduced.
• In Fanconi's anaemia lymphocyte chromosomes show random breaks.

Specific therapy
• Immunosuppression, e.g. antilymphocyte globulin (ALG), horse or rabbit, given intravenously over several days, corticosteroids and cyclosporin (alone or with ALG) improve marrow function in 50–70% of severe cases.
• Androgens (e.g. oxymetholone) may benefit Fanconi's anaemia and acquired aplastic anaemia.
• Bone marrow transplantation offers a cure in severe cases, providing there is an HLA matching sibling to act as

donor. Results are best (60–70% cure) in younger patients (<20 years).
• Haemopoietic growth factors, granulocyte colony-stimulating factor or granulocyte-macrophage colony-stimulating factor may raise the neutrophil count temporarily but have no long-term benefit on the underlying bone marrow defect.
• Blood product support (Chapter 37).

Red cell aplasia
Red cell aplasia is anaemia caused by selective reduction of red cell production by the bone marrow. There is absence or severe reduction of developing erythroblasts in the marrow and of reticulocytes in the peripheral blood, with no abnormality in other cell lines.

Clinical and laboratory features
A rare congenital form (Diamond–Blackfan anaemia) is frequently associated with other somatic malformations. Acquired red cell aplasia may occur as a result of drugs (e.g. azathioprine, isoniazid), in association with autoimmune diseases (e.g. systemic lupus erythematosus), haematological malignancy (e.g. chronic lymphocytic leukaemia) or with a thymoma (see Chapter 34).

Transient red cell aplasia occurs following infection with B19 parvovirus and can lead to a profound but temporary reduction of red cell production with severe anaemia in patients with a haemolytic disorder (e.g. 'aplastic crisis' in hereditary spherocytosis or sickle cell anaemia).

Treatment
Treatment of the underlying disorder (e.g. removal of a thymoma) is required. Red cell transfusion and iron chelation therapy may be required. Immunosuppressive therapy (e.g. prednisolone, cyclosporin, ALG) is useful in selected patients with either congenital or acquired red cell aplasia.

Congenital dyserythopoietic anaemias
Congenital dyserythropoietic anaemias are a rare group of recessively inherited conditions in which chronic anaemia results from abnormal maturation of erythroid cells in the marrow. Red cell precursors usually show marked morphological abnormalities, e.g. bi- and trinucleated normoblasts.

19 Haematological malignancy: basic mechanisms

Neoplasia

Haematological malignancies (Table 19.1) are thought to arise from a single cell in the bone marrow, thymus or peripheral lymphoid system. This cell undergoes genetic change (mutation) leading to malignant *transformation*. Successive mitotic divisions give rise to a clone of cells derived from the parent cell. Further mutations may give rise to subclones (clonal evolution). Transformed cells either proliferate excessively or are resistant to apoptosis. They are often 'frozen' at a particular stage of differentiation.

Causes of neoplasia

Neoplasia is caused by a complex interaction between genetic and environmental mechanisms (Fig. 19.1).

1 Genetic predisposition. Certain inherited conditions (e.g. Down's syndrome, trisomy 21) and conditions associated with defective DNA repair (e.g. Fanconi's anaemia) or immune suppression (e.g. ataxia telangiectasia).
2 Viral infection. Human T-cell leukaemia virus (HTLV-1) incorporates into T-lymphoid-cell genome and underlies adult T-cell leukaemia lymphoma (see Chapter 26). Other viruses predispose to malignancy by immune suppression (e.g. HIV). Epidemiological evidence implicates Epstein–Barr virus in Burkitt's lymphoma.
3 Ionizing radiation causes DNA mutation and increases the risk of haematological neoplasia.
4 Toxins/chemicals, e.g. benzene and organochemicals may predispose to leukaemia and myelodysplasia (MDS).
5 Drugs. Alkylating agents (e.g. melphalan, mustine)

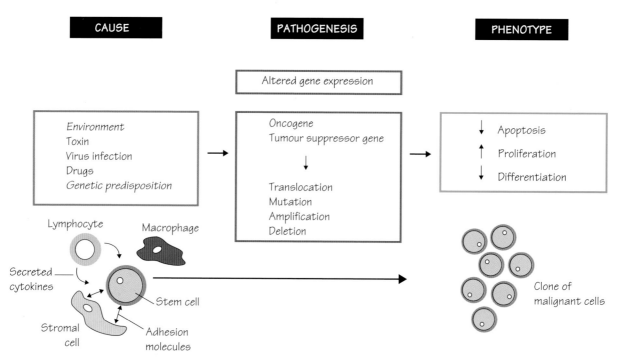

Fig. 19.1 Pathogenesis of haematological malignancy.

Table 19.1 Classification of haematological malignancies.

	Acute	Chronic
Lymphoid	Acute lymphoblastic leukaemia (ALL) and subtypes	Chronic lymphocytic leukaemia (CLL) and variants Non-Hodgkin lymphoma (NHL) Hodgkin lymphoma (HL) Multiple myeloma and variants
Myeloid	Acute myeloid leukaemia (AML) and subtypes	Chronic myeloid leukaemia (CML) and variants Myelodysplasia (MDS) Myeloproliferative disorders

and other forms of chemotherapy predispose to MDS or acute myeloid leukaemia.

Mechanism of malignant transformation
Altered expression of three types of gene underlies multistep pathogenesis of haematological malignancy.

1 Oncogenes
These are genes whose protein products cause neoplastic transformation. Oncogenes are derived from normal cellular genes (proto-oncogenes) which code for proteins usually involved in one or other stage in cell signal transduction, gene transcription, cell cycle, cell survival/ apoptosis or differentiation. Inappropriate activation and expression of an oncogene may cause transformation. Activation of oncogenes may occur by **amplification**, **point mutation** or **translocation** (most frequent in haematological malignancies) from one chromosomal location to another. Translocation may lead to a quantitative change in expression (e.g. MYC translocation to the immunoglobulin heavy chain locus in lymphoid neoplasia, t(8;14)) or qualitative change by joining all or part of the oncogene to another gene to form a fusion gene (e.g. ABL translocation to the breakpoint cluster region [BCR] to form BCR-ABL in CML, t[9;22]).

2 Anti-oncogenes
Anti-oncogenes, or tumour suppressor genes (e.g. *p53*), are genes encoding proteins which have a critical role in suppressing cell growth. Chromosome deletion may obliterate tumour suppressor genes on one allele; deletion or mutation of the remaining allele may allow uncontrolled cell growth.

3 Inhibition of apoptosis
Malignant cells often show resistance to apoptosis. The BCL-2 gene product inhibits apoptosis and its expression is increased in some chromosome translocations (e.g. in follicular lymphoma).

Evidence of clonality
A population of cells is considered clonal (derived from a single cell by mitotic division) if they have some or all the following.
• The same acquired chromosome abnormality, e.g. Ph chromosome (see Fig. 20.1) or point mutation within an individual gene.
• Clonal rearrangement of an immunoglobulin or T cell receptor gene in lymphoid neoplasia.
• Restriction in a B-lymphoid neoplasm to expression of only λ or κ light chains, but not both as in polyclonal B cells.
• Restriction fragment length polymorphism in which the size of a restriction fragment of DNA on the X chromo-

some is analysed. In females, two fragments derived from the two X chromosomes will be found in polyclonal populations, both fragments being transcriptionally active and hypomethylated. In tumours only one size of fragment is hypomethylated as only one X chromosome is active.

Minimal residual disease (Fig. 19.2)
At the time of diagnosis of a haematological neoplasm, the patient will have approximately 10^{13}–10^{14} malignant cells. Even if treatment results in 1000-fold reduction of tumour cells, there remain 10^{10} cells, which may be below the conventional level of detection. Using immunological or molecular techniques, residual malignant cells may be detected in blood or marrow of patients who clinically and by conventional light microscopy are in complete remission.

Techniques
These techniques (see Chapter 7) include:
• immunological, particularly if residual malignant cells carry a distinctively abnormal phenotype;
• chromosomal analysis and FISH (p. 27); and
• molecular using the polymerase chain reaction, which are the most sensitive (will detect one malignant cell in up to 10^6 normal cells).

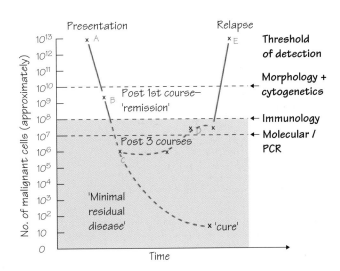

Fig. 19.2 Minimal residual disease. Morphologically obvious disease (e.g. in AML) is present at presentation (A). At remission (B), when there is no morphological evidence of disease, there are still substantial numbers of malignant cells and disease is detectable by immunological and molecular techniques. At (C) there is no disease detectable, but there may well be minimal residual disease. At (D) disease is once more detectable and, in this example, precedes overt relapse.

20 Chronic myeloid leukaemia

This is a clonal myeloproliferative disorder characterized by an increase in neutrophils and their precursors in the peripheral blood with increased cellularity of the marrow as a result of an excess of granulocyte precursors. The leukaemic cells of >95% of patients have a reciprocal translocation between the long arms of chromosomes 9 and 22, t(9;22). The derived chromosome 22 is termed the Philadelphia (Ph) chromosome (Fig. 20.1). The disease usually transforms from a relatively stable chronic phase to an acute leukaemia phase (blast transformation).

Aetiology and pathophysiology
Aetiology is unknown. Exposure to ionizing radiation is a risk factor. The ABL oncogene is translocated from chromosome 9 into the breakpoint cluster region (BCR) on chromosome 22 to form the BCR-ABL fusion gene (see Fig. 20.1) This fusion gene encodes a 210-kDa protein with greatly increased tyrosine kinase activity compared to the normal ABL product. The disease is of stem cell origin as the Ph chromosome is present in erythroid, granulocytic, megakaryocytic and T-lymphoid precursors. Rare cases show variant translocations, or are Ph-negative but show the BCR-ABL fusion gene. The Ph chromosome abnormality may also occur in acute lymphoblastic leukaemia (ALL; see Chapter 22).

Clinical features
• Occurs at all ages (peak age 25–45 years, male/female ratio equal, incidence of 5–10 cases/million population).
• Patients usually present in the chronic phase.
• Presenting symptoms include weight loss, night sweats, itching, left hypochondrial pain, gout.
• Priapism, visual disturbance and headaches caused by hyperviscosity (WBC>250×10^9/L) are less frequent.
• Splenomegaly, often massive, occurs in over 90% of cases.
• Some cases are discovered on routine blood test.

Laboratory findings
• Raised white cell count (often 50×10^9/L or more), mainly neutrophils and myelocytes (Fig. 20.2).
• Basophils may be prominent.
• Platelet count may be raised, normal or low and anaemia may be present.
• Low leucocyte alkaline phosphatase score, raised serum B_{12} and B_{12}-binding protein (transcobalamin I).

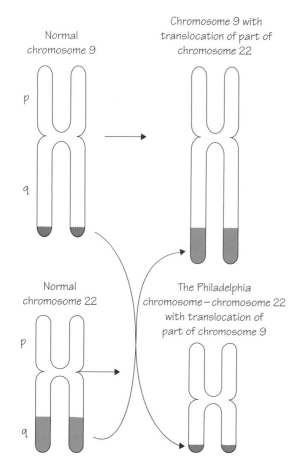

Normal chromosome 9

Chromosome 9 with translocation of part of chromosome 22

p

q

Normal chromosome 22

The Philadelphia chromosome – chromosome 22 with translocation of part of chromosome 9

p

q

Fig. 20.1 The Philadelphia chromosome is an abnormal chromosome 22 caused by translocation of part of long arm (q) of chromosome 22 to chromosome 9, and reciprocal translocation of part of chromosome 9, including the ABL oncogene, to a specific breakpoint cluster region (BCR) of chromosome 22. A fusion gene results on the derived chromosome 22 which leads to the synthesis of an abnormal protein with tyrosine protein kinase activity that is much greater than that of the normal ABL protein.

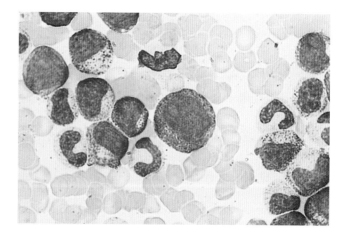

Fig. 20.2 Chronic myeloid leukaemia (chronic phase): peripheral blood film, showing immature granulocytes (myelocytes, metamyelocytes) in the peripheral blood.

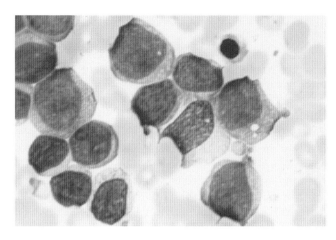

Fig. 20.3 Chronic myeloid leukaemia: blast transformation. There is replacement by homogenous blast cells.

• Raised serum uric acid.

• Bone marrow is hypercellular with a raised myeloid/ erythroid ratio (see Chapter 1).

• Cytogenetic analysis of bone marrow cells shows the Philadelphia chromosome in >95% of metaphases. The BCR-ABL fusion gene is detectable by FISH (see p. 27) and its RNA product by PCR (see p. 28).

Course and progress

Patients are typically well during the 'chronic phase'. Main cause of death is transformation into acute leukaemia (Fig. 20.3) (80% AML, 20% ALL, with a proportion showing a mixed blast cell population), which may occur at any stage, even at presentation. Median survival is currently about 4 years. Staging to predict prognosis has been attempted using age, spleen size, blood blast cell and platelet counts.

There may be an accelerated phase in which anaemia, thrombocytopenia, splenic enlargement and marrow fibrosis occur. Transformation is usually accompanied by additional morphological and chromosome abnormalities.

Treatment

Chronic phase

• Hydroxyurea will control the raised white cell count.

• α-interferon (IFN) may also control the white cell count and may delay onset of acute transformation, prolonging overall survival by 1–2 years. The best responders to IFN become Ph-negative, but usually remain BCR-ABL-positive, and have the best prognosis, but must continue IFN. Combination therapies, e.g. IFN + cytosine arabinoside, may be more effective than IFN alone.

• Allopurinol to prevent hyperuricaemia.

• Allogeneic stem cell transplantation (SCT) before the age of 50 from an HLA matching sibling offers a 70% chance of cure in chronic phase but 30% or less once acceleration has occurred. HLA-matched unrelated donor (MUD) SCT is less successful in curing the disease because of higher morbidity and mortality. Transfusion of donor lymphocytes may be valuable in eliminating BCR-ABL-positive cells in case of relapse post-SCT.

• A specific inhibitor (STI 571) of the tyrosine kinase encoded by BCR-ABL causes the marrow to become Ph negative in a high proportion of cases and may improve the treatment of CML. This drug may also be of benefit in patients with Ph +ve ALL.

Acute phase

Therapy as for acute leukaemia, AML or ALL may be given, but the prognosis is poor. The value of STI 571 is under trial.

21 Myelodysplasia

This is a clonal disorder of the haemopoietic stem cell characterized by peripheral blood cytopenias affecting more than one lineage in association with a cellular marrow, indicating ineffective haempoiesis.

Aetiology and pathogenesis

Myelodysplasia (MDS) may be primary (*de novo*) or a consequence of previous chemotherapy/radiotherapy (secondary). Various chromosome and oncogene abnormalities occur, e.g. complete or partial deletions of chromosomes 5 or 7, point mutations in RAS oncogenes. The disease is divided into five subgroups (Table 21.1). It may transform to acute myeloid leukaemia (AML) (>30% blasts in the marrow).

Clinical features

• Most frequent in the elderly but young adults or even children may be affected.
• Bone marrow failure (see Chapter 18) with anaemia and/or leucopenia and/or thrombocytopenia.
• In chronic myelomonocytic leukaemia (CMML), the spleen may be enlarged.
• The 5q-syndrome is a subgroup, occurring particularly in elderly females with a high platelet count, macrocytosis and good prognosis.

Laboratory findings

• Anaemia is usually macrocytic.
• Neutropenia is frequent and neutrophils may be hypogranular with pseudo-Pelger forms (Fig. 21.1). Monocytes are increased in CMML to >1.0×10^9/L.
• Bone marrow is usually hypercellular but may be hypocellular and/or fibrotic.

• Characteristic morphological changes are seen in all three lineages (Figs 21.1–21.4).

Differential diagnosis

This is very broad, particularly when only one lineage is involved in an elderly person. Thus, other causes of anaemia, e.g. haematinic deficiency, renal disease, hypothyroidism, anaemia of chronic disease must be excluded; some or all may coexist with MDS. Thrombocytopenia or leucopenia may be caused by drugs, immune destruction or hypersplenism. The hallmark of MDS is involvement of more than one—typically all three—lineage(s). Nevertheless, distinction between MDS, myelofibrosis and aplasia may be difficult in patients with pancytopenia. The finding of a cytogenetic abnormality greatly strengthens what may otherwise be a subjective morphological diagnosis.

Course and prognosis

This depends on the type of MDS (see Table 21.1). The degree of cytopenia influences the incidence of complications and treatment, while the percentage of blast cells is predictive of the risk of developing acute leukaemia. The presence of complex cytogenetic changes is also associated with a poor prognosis. Scoring systems have been devised whereby the degree of cytopenia, proportion of blasts and nature of cytogenetic changes is used to estimate prognosis. Death may be caused by infection, haemorrhage, iron overload from multiple transfusions or from transformation into AML.

Treatment

• Support care with red cell or platelet transfusions and antimicrobials may be required.

Table 21.1 Classification of the myelodysplastic syndromes.

Disease	Peripheral blood	Bone marrow	Approximate median survival (months)
1 Refractory anaemia*	Blasts <1%	Blasts <5%	50
2 RA with ring sideroblasts	Blasts <1%	Blasts <5% Ring sideroblasts >15% of total erythroblasts	50
3 RAEB	Blasts <5%	Blasts 5–20%	11
4 RAEB-t	Blasts >5%	Blasts 20–30% or Auer rods present	5
5 CMML	As any of the above with >1.0×10^9/L monocytes	As any of the above with promonocytes	11

* In some cases neutropenia or thrombocytopenia is present without anaemia. These cases are termed refractory anaemia.
CMML, chronic myelomonocytic leukaemia; RA, refractory anaemia; RAEB, RA with excess blasts; RAEB-t, RAEB in transformation.

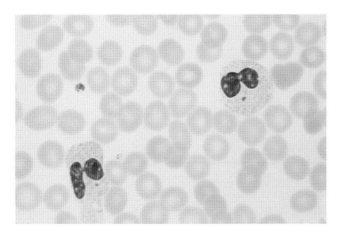

Fig. 21.1 Myelodysplasia: peripheral blood film showing hypogranular neutrophils with bi-lobed nuclei (pseudo-Pelger cells).

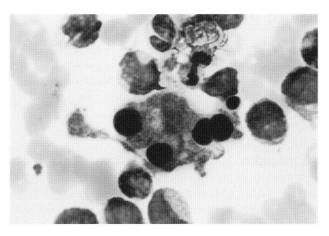

Fig. 21.3 Myelodysplasia: bone marrow aspirate showing mononuclear and binuclear micromegakaryocytes.

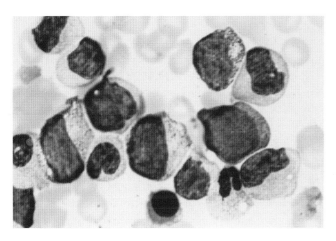

Fig. 21.2 Myelodysplasia: bone marrow aspirate showing a granular bast with blue cytoplasm and hypogranular maturing myeloid cells.

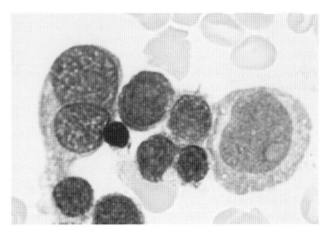

Fig. 21.4 Myelodysplasia: bone marrow aspirate showing an erythroblast and abnormal normoblast (dyserythropoiesis). Ringed sideroblasts (see Fig. 10.3) may also occur.

• Iron chelation therapy may be needed for multiply transfused iron loaded patients with an otherwise good prognosis.

• Granulocyte colony-stimulating factor (G-CSF) or granulocyte-macrophage colony-stimulating factor (GM-CSF) may be used temporarily to increase neutrophil and monocyte production; erythropoietin produces a rise in haemoglobin in about 5–15% of patients with RA.

• Chemotherapy with low-dose ara-C, etoposide, thioguanine or 6-mercaptopurine is used to control excess blast proliferation in patients unsuitable for high-dose chemotherapy.

• Younger patients with refractory anaemia with excess blasts (RAEB) and RAEB in transformation (RAEB-t) may be treated as AML. Fludarabine, ara-C, G-CSF ± idarubicin (FLAG ±Ida) is a useful form of combination chemotherapy. Complete remissions are less frequent than in *de novo* AML. Allogeneic SCT (sibling or MUD) may cure younger patients.

Acute leukaemia is a malignant disorder in which haemopoietic blast cells constitute >30% of bone marrow cells. The primitive cells usually also accumulate in the blood, infiltrate other tissues and cause bone marrow failure.

Classification

There are two main groups: acute lymphoblastic (ALL); and acute myeloid (myeloblastic) leukaemia (AML). Rare cases are undifferentiated or mixed. Subclassification of ALL or AML depends on morphological, immunological, cytochemical and cytogenetic criteria (Tables 22.1–22.3).

Aetiology and pathogenesis

The malignant cells typically show a chromosome translocation or other DNA mutation affecting oncogenes and anti-oncogenes (see Chapter 19). AML may follow previous myeloproliferative or myelodysplastic diseases. In childhood B lineage (common) ALL there is evidence that the first event, a chromosomal translocation, may occur *in utero* and subsequent events (? infection) precipitate the onset of ALL.

Incidence

Approximately 1000 new cases (20–25/million population) each of AML and ALL per year in the UK. ALL is the most common malignancy in childhood (peak age 4 years) but also occurs in adults. AML occurs at all ages but is rarer than ALL in childhood, being most common in the elderly.

Clinical features

• Short (<3-month) history of symptoms due to bone marrow failure (e.g. anaemia, abnormal bruising/bleeding or infection). Disseminated intravascular coagulation (DIC) with bleeding is particularly common in AML M3.
• Increased cellular catabolism may cause sweating, fever and general malaise.
• Lymphadenopathy and hepatosplenomegaly are frequent, especially in ALL.
• Tissue infiltration, e.g. of meninges, testes (more common in ALL), skin, bones, gums with hypertrophy (AML M5 or M4) may cause clinical symptoms or signs.

Laboratory features

• Anaemia, thrombocytopenia and often neutropenia.
• Leucocytosis caused by blast cells in the blood usually occurs. Leucopenia is less frequent.
• The bone marrow shows infiltration by blast cells (>30% and often 80–90% of marrow cells).
• Coagulation may be abnormal and DIC can occur, especially with AML M3.
• Serum uric acid, lactate dehydrogenase (LDH) may be raised.
• Morphological analysis (Figs 22.1–22.12, Table 22.1) usually reveals cytoplasmic granules or Auer rods (condensations of granules) in AML. Cytochemical stains are helpful—AML blasts have granules positive by Sudan black, myeloperoxidase and chloroacetate esterase, while monoblasts are positive for non-specific and butyrate esterase. B-lineage lymphoblasts show blocks of positive material with periodic acid–Schiff (PAS) stain, and in T-lineage ALL with acid phosphatase.
• Immunophenotype analysis involves use of antibodies to identify cell antigens (many termed clusters of differentiation or CD, see Appendix I) which correlate with lineage and maturity (Table 22.2). Other antigens, e.g. TdT, and cytoplasmic immunoglobulin may be also be detected.
• Cytogenetic analysis gives diagnostic and prognostic information (Tables 22.3 and 22.4).

Table 22.1 French–American–British (FAB) classification of acute leukaemia.

Myeloid	Lymphoid
M0 Undifferentiated by morphology + cytochemistry, myeloid immunophenotype	L1 Small cells, high nuclear/cytoplasmic ratio
M1 Little differentiation, >90% blasts	L2 Larger cells, lower nuclear/cytoplasmic ratio
M2 Differentiated, 30–90% blasts	L3 Vacuolated, basophilic blast cells
M3 Promyelocytic: intensely granular, variant form is microgranular	
M4 Myelomonocytic	
M5a Monocytic without differentiation	
M5b Monocytic with differentiation	
M6 Erythroid differentiation, >50% of mononuclear cells are erythroid	
M7 Megakaryoblastic	

* All subtypes have >30% blast cells in the bone marrow.

Table 22.2 Immunophenotypes of acute leukaemia.

Disease	Immunophenotype
AML	CD33, CD13
	Monocytic cells: CD14, CD61
	Megakaryoblasts: CD41, CD61
	Erythroid: glycophorin, transferrin receptor (CD71)
ALL	
Early B-precursors (Pro-B)	CD19, TdT
Common ALL	CD10, CD19, cyt CD22, TdT
Pre B-ALL	cyIg, CD19, cyt CD22, TdT
B-ALL	sMIg, CD19, CD20
T-ALL	CD7, cyt CD3, TdT

CD34 is a marker of haemopoietic stem cells and may be positive in both AML and ALL.
ALL, acute lymphoblastic leukaemia; AML, acute myeloid leukaemia; B-ALL, B cell ALL; CyIg, cytoplasmic immunoglobin; sMIg, surface membrane immunoglobulin; T-ALL, T cell ALL; TdT, terminal deoxynucleotidyl transferase.

Table 22.3 Cytogenetic changes in acute myeloid leukaemia.

Good risk

M2: t(8,21)
M3: t(15,17)
M4 eosinophilia: inversion 16

Poor risk

Monosomy 5, monosomy 7
Complex karyotypes
11q 23 abnormalities
Mutation of FLt-3

Standard risk

All other cases

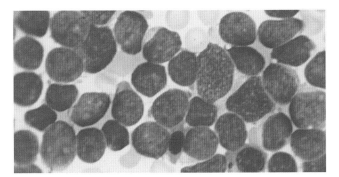

Fig. 22.1 T-cell acute lymphoblastic leukaemia (T-ALL): bone marrow showing large numbers of lymphoblasts with a high nuclear/cytoplasmic ratio.

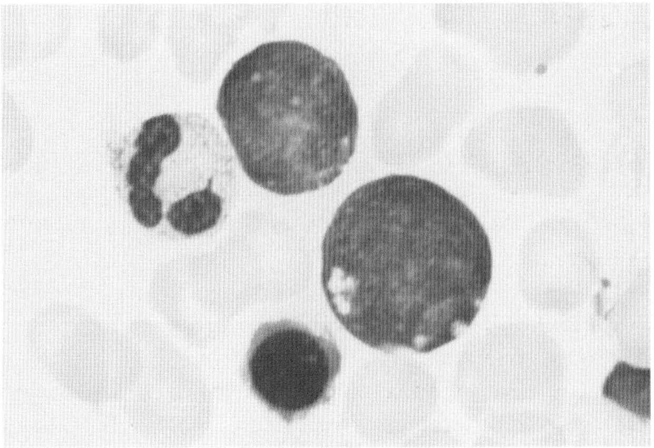

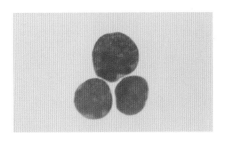

Fig. 22.2 B-cell ALL: bone marrow showing large blasts with characteristic vacuoles and blue cytoplasm.

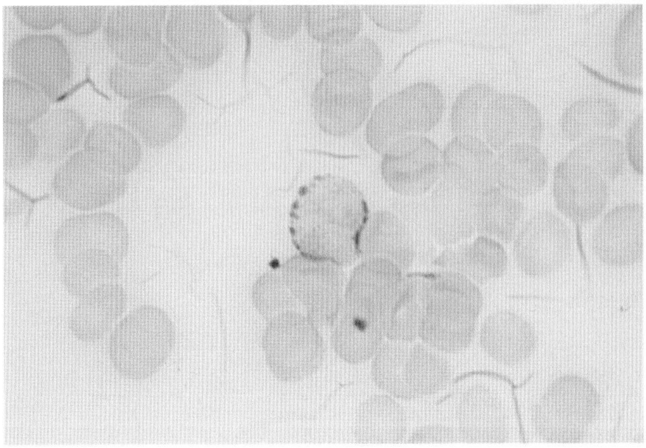

Fig. 22.3 Common ALL: bone marrow—periodic acid–Schiff stain showing block positivity in blast cells.

Fig. 22.4 Common ALL: cerebrospinal fluid cytocentrifuge specimen showing lymphoblasts.

Treatment

The first phase of therapy (remission-induction) is with high-dose intensive combination chemotherapy to reduce or eradicate leukaemic cells from the bone marrow and re-establish normal haemopoiesis. Further therapy is postinduction chemotherapy: this may be intensive ('intensification' or 'consolidation' chemotherapy) or less intensive

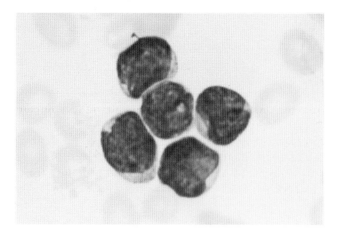

Fig. 22.5 Acute myeloid leukaemia: bone marrow—M0.

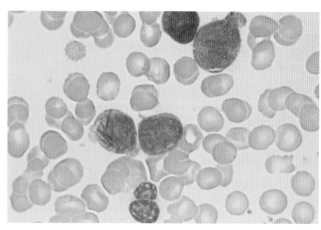

Fig. 22.8 Acute myeloid leukaemia: bone marrow—M3. Note cell with multiple Auer rods.

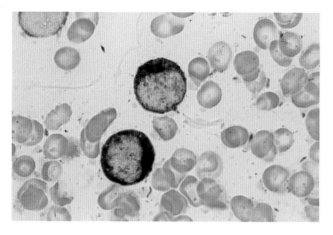

Fig. 22.6 Acute myeloid leukaemia: bone marrow—M1 (Sudan black stain, showing primary granules).

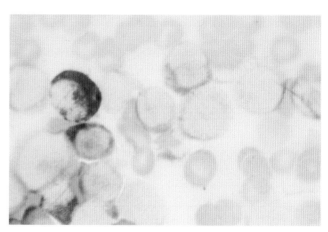

Fig. 22.9 Acute myeloid leukaemia: bone marrow—M4. Combined esterase stain, showing myeloblasts (blue) and monoblasts (brown).

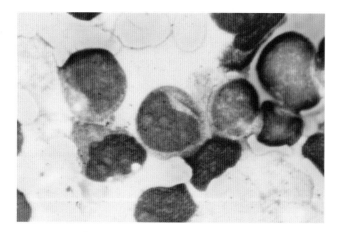

Fig. 22.7 Acute myeloid leukaemia: bone marrow—M2. Note Auer rod in myeloblast.

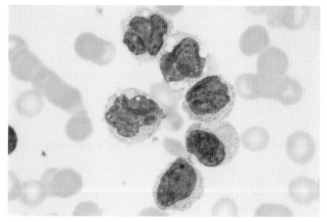

Fig. 22.10 Acute myeloid leukaemia: bone marrow—M5. Showing vacuolated monoblasts.

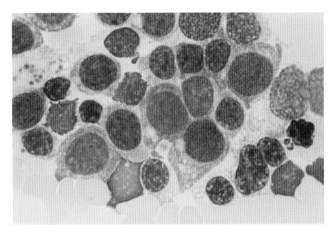

Fig. 22.11 Acute myeloid leukaemia: bone marrow—M6. Showing abnormal erythroid cells, erythroblasts and myeloblasts.

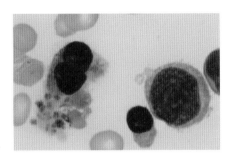

Fig. 22.12 Acute myeloid leukaemia: bone marrow—M7. Showing myeloblasts and megakaryoblasts, with platelets budding from the cytoplasm.

Table 22.4 Prognostic factors in acute lymphoblastic leukaemia.

	Good	Bad
Sex	Female	Male
Age	2–9 years	Adult
White cell count	Low (<10×10⁹/L)	High (>50×10⁹/L)
Chromosomes	Hyperdiploid	t(9;22), t(4;11)
Extramedullary disease	Absent	Present
Speed of remission	4 weeks	>4 weeks
Clearance of peripheral blood blasts	1 week	>1 week
Loss of minimal residual disease in bone marrow	1–3 months	>3 months

(maintenance chemotherapy). Each course of intensive treatment typically requires 4–6 weeks in hospital.

Acute myeloid leukaemia

Remission induction regimes usually comprise an anthracycline (e.g. daunorubicin), cytosine arabinoside and etoposide or thioguanine. All trans retinoic acid (ATRA) is given concurrently in AML M3 to induce differentiation. More than 80% of patients under the age of 60 years achieve remission, defined as a normal full blood count and film with <5% blasts in bone marrow, with one course and >85% with two courses. Older patients and those with preceding MDS or AML secondary to another disease (e.g. myeloproliferative disorder, MPD) have lower remission rates. Three or four further courses are given as post-induction therapy, and other agents used include mitoxantrone, M-AMSA, idarubicin and high dose ara-c. Tumour lysis syndrome may occur (see p. 108).

Acute lymphoblastic leukaemia

Remission induction regimes comprise vincristine, prednisolone and L-asparaginase often with daunorubicin, cyclophosphamide. Post-remission therapy is with two or three 'intensification' blocks with additional drugs. Patients then receive maintenance chemotherapy for a further 2 to 3 years with daily mercaptopurine, weekly methotrexate and monthly vincristine and prednisolone.

Central nervous system involvement is common in ALL in children and adults, and normal practice is to give multiple intrathecal injections and courses of high-dose systemic chemotherapy with methotrexate or cranial radiotherapy to prevent or treat this complication.

Stem cell transplantation (see Chapter 38)

Allogeneic stem cell transplantation (SCT) is usually recommended for patients (<50 years) in first remission of AML and for adults with ALL (>20 years, <50 years) who have a histocompatible sibling. Good prognosis AML (Table 22.3) and ALL (Table 22.4) cases are not given SCT in first remission. Autologous peripheral blood stem cell transplant (PBSCT) in some studies has improved cure rate compared to chemotherapy alone in AML and adult ALL in first or subsequent remission.

Complications of chemotherapy and supportive care are considered in Chapter 39; blood component therapy is considered in Chapter 37.

Prognosis

Childhood acute lymphoblastic leukaemia

Overall 70% of children with ALL are cured, the best responses being in girls, aged 2–12 years with low presenting white cell count (<10×10⁹/L) and favourable cytogenetics (Table 22.4).

Acute myeloid leukaemia and adult acute lymphoblastic leukaemia

Approximately 30–40% of patients are cured but this varies widely according to age and prognostic features.

23 Chronic lymphocytic leukaemia

Chronic lymphocytic leukaemia (CLL) is a B-cell clonal lymphoproliferative disease in which lymphocytes accumulate in the blood, bone marrow and often in the lymph nodes and spleen (absolute lymphocyte count $> 5.0 \times 10^9$/L). A disease of older patients (peak age 72), it is the commonest leukaemia in Western countries (over 70 new cases/million population/year in the UK, male/female ratio 2 : 1) but is rare in Asia.

Aetiology and pathophysiology

The cause is unknown. Commonest chromosome changes are trisomy 12, a 13q deletion and deletions of 11q including the ataxia telangiectasia gene. Oncogene mutations or deletions occur which may prevent cells from undergoing programmed cell death (apoptosis).

Clinical features

Stages depend on clinical and laboratory findings (Fig. 23.1).
• Many cases (Stage A) are symptomless and diagnosed on routine blood test.
• Presenting features include lymphadenopathy (typically symmetrical, painless and discrete), night sweats, loss of weight, symptoms of bone marrow failure.
• Spleen is often moderately enlarged.
• Hypogammaglobulinaemia and reduced cell-mediated immunity predispose to bacterial and viral infection.

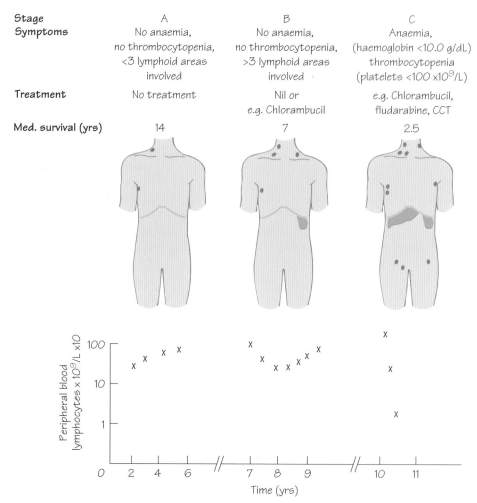

Stage	A	B	C
Symptoms	No anaemia, no thrombocytopenia, <3 lymphoid areas involved	No anaemia, no thrombocytopenia, >3 lymphoid areas involved	Anaemia, (haemoglobin <10.0 g/dL) thrombocytopenia (platelets <100 x10⁹/L)
Treatment	No treatment	Nil or e.g. Chlorambucil	e.g. Chlorambucil, fludarabine, CCT
Med. survival (yrs)	14	7	2.5

Fig. 23.1 The clinical course of chronic lymphocytic leukaemia (CLL). The Binet staging system evaluates enlargement of the following: lymph nodes, whether unilateral or bilateral, in the head and neck, axillae and inguinal regions; spleen and liver. Stage A patients are usually asymptomatic and do not require treatment. The peripheral blood lymphocyte count may rise progressively. Stage B patients often require treatment (e.g. with oral chlorambucil). Stage C patients will often respond to more intensive therapy (fludarabine, combination chemotherapy (CCT)).

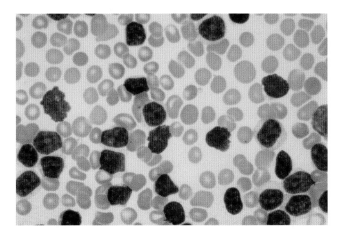

Fig. 23.2 Chronic lymphocytic leukaemia: peripheral blood film showing large numbers of mature lymphoid cells and some 'smear' cells.

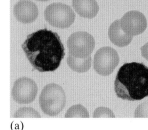
(a)

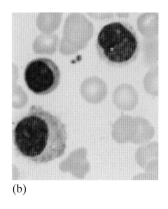
(b)

Fig. 23.3 (a) Prolymphocytic leukaemia: blood film. (b) Hairy cell leukaemia: blood film.

Laboratory findings
• Increased peripheral blood lymphocytes (Fig. 23.2 usually $10–30 \times 10^9/L$ at presentation) which are B cells (CD19, CD22 and also CD5 positive).
• They have weak expression of surface IgM which is monoclonal (expressing only κ or only λ light chains).
• Serum immunoglobulins are depressed.
• Anaemia and thrombocytopenia may occur due to marrow infiltration or as a result of auto-antibodies.

Course and prognosis
Patients may present at an early stage and subsequently remain stationary, progress or may present with late-stage disease. Some patients need no treatment for 10 years or more whilst in others the disease follows an aggressive course. Local immunoblastic transformation (Richter's syndrome) may be a terminal event. The natural history correlates with the maturity of the cell of origin, post-germinal centre (good) or pre-germinal centre (bad).

Treatment
• Observation only for asymptomatic Stage A patients.
• Oral chlorambucil to lower the lymphocyte count and reduce lymph node and spleen size.
• Corticosteroids for bone marrow failure due to infiltration and for autoimmune haemolytic anaemia or thrombocytopenia.

• The purine analogue fludarabine is valuable, either alone or in combination.
• Combination chemotherapy e.g. CHOP (see Chapter 26).
• Support care (Chapter 39).
• Splenectomy or splenic irradiation is useful if the spleen is large and causes local symptoms or as a result of hypersplenism.

Variants of chronic lymphocytic leukaemia
Prolymphocytic leukaemia (PLL, Fig. 23.3a) resembles CLL but usually occurs in older (> 70 years) patients, the white cell count is high and responds poorly to treatment.

Hairy cell leukaemia (HCL, Fig. 23.3b) is rare (male/female ratio of 4 : 1, peak age of 55 years), presents with splenomegaly and pancytopenia. 'Hairy cells' are present in bone marrow and blood. Infections are frequent. They are B cells which stain for tartrate resistant acid phosphatase. Effective treatments include 2-chloro-deoxyadenosine (2-CDA) deoxycoformycin, interferon-α and splenectomy.

T-cell variants of CLL, PLL and HCL are much rarer than B-cell type and are more aggressive.

Leukaemia/lymphoma syndromes. Circulating lymphoma cells may occur in different non-Hodgkin lymphomas, e.g. follicular lymphoma, mantle cell lymphoma, lymphoplasmacytoid lymphoma and adult T-cell leukaemia/lymphoma.

24 Multiple myeloma

Multiple myeloma (MM) is a malignant disorder of plasma cells characterized by:
1 a monoclonal paraprotein in serum and/or urine;
2 bone changes leading to pain and pathological features;
3 excess plasma cells in the bone marrow.

Incidence
Approximately 50 cases/million population; 15% of lymphoid malignancies; 2% of all malignancies; twice as common in black than white people; slightly more common in males than females; median age at diagnosis 71 years.

Aetiology and pathogenesis
The aetiology is unknown. The cell of origin is probably a postgerminal centre B-lymphoid cell. The cells all secrete the same immunoglobulin (Ig) or Ig component, e.g. part of a heavy chain attached to a light chain or light chain (κ or λ) alone. Rarely (<1%) the cells are non-secretory. Interleukin-6 (IL-6) from myeloma cells themselves or accessory cells promotes plasma cell growth. Tumour necrosis factor (TNF) and IL-1 mediate bone resorption. Oncogene mutations (e.g. *ras*, p53, *myc*) and translocations to 14q occur. Chromosomal deletions of 13q generally imply a poor prognosis.

Clinical features
• Skeletal involvement—bone pain, especially lower backache, or pathological fracture.
• Marrow infiltration—features of bone marrow failure.
• Infection—lack of normal immunoglobulins (immune paresis) and neutropenia.
• Renal failure occurs in up to one-third of patients and is caused by hypercalcaemia, infection, deposition of paraprotein or light chains, uric acid or amyloid.
• Amyloidosis may cause macroglossia, hepatosplenomegaly, cardiac or renal failure, carpal tunnel syndrome and autonomic neuropathy.

Laboratory features
• Anaemia is frequent, often with neutropenia and thrombocytopenia. Erythrocyte sedimentation rate (ESR) often >100 mm/h.
• Blood film shows rouleaux with a bluish background staining, caused by the protein increase. Leuco-erythroblastic picture may be present.
• Bone marrow shows >10% plasma cells, often with multinucleate and other abnormal forms (Fig. 24.1).
• A paraprotein in serum and/or Bence Jones protein (light chains) in urine with suppression of normal serum immunoglobulins is usual (Fig. 24.2).

• The paraprotein is IgG in 70%; IgA in 20%; IgM is uncommon; IgD and IgE are rare.
• Serum β_2 microglobulin (β_2M) often raised and higher levels correlate with worse prognosis.
• Serum alkaline phosphatase usually normal.
• X-rays, CT scan or MRI show lytic lesions typically in skull and axial skeleton and/or osteoporosis, often with pathological fractures (Fig. 24.3). Occasional patients show localized plasma cell deposits, typically in the axial skeleton (multiple or solitary plasmacytoma).
• Prognostic data include haemoglobin level, serum levels of β_2M, serum creatinine and extent of skeletal disease.

Treatment
• Symptomless patients who are stable with normal blood counts and renal function, no skeletal disease and low levels of paraprotein warrant observation rather than therapy.
• Chemotherapy: induction is usually with melphalan and prednisolone or combination chemotherapy, e.g. Adriamycin, BCNU, cyclophosphamide and melphalan (ABCM) given intermittently every 4–6 weeks.
• Most patients will reach a stable (plateau) phase (clinically well with near normal blood count, <5% plasma cells in bone marrow, stable paraprotein level) after 4–6 cycles of treatment. This lasts 1–3 years. α-Interferon may prolong duration of plateau phase.
• Intensive therapy, e.g. slow infusions of vincristine, Adriamycin and dexamethasone (VAD), more often (>50%) leads to complete disappearance of paraprotein and normalization of blood and marrow morphology (complete remission).
• Younger patients (<60 years) may benefit from induction with courses of VAD followed by high-dose chemotherapy,

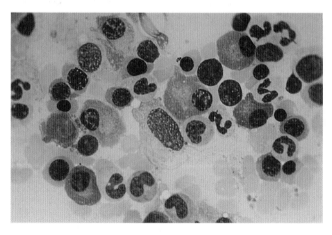

Fig. 24.1 Multiple myeloma: bone marrow showing infiltration by plasma cells.

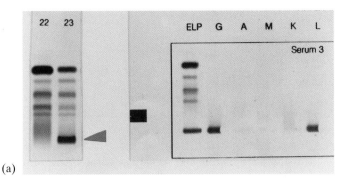

(a)

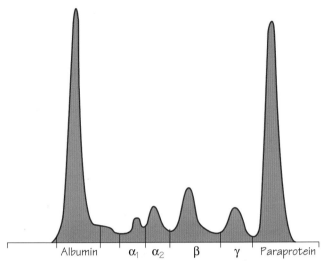

Protein electrophoresis

(b)

Name	%	g/L	Normal (g/L)
Albumin	27.2	24.8	35 – 47
Gammaglobulin	2.1	1.9	25 – 33
Paraprotein	47.6	43.4	

Fig. 24.2 Multiple myeloma: protein electrophoresis. (a) Lane 22 shows a normal patient. Patient 23 has a paraprotein. The panel on the right shows that this paraprotein reacts with IgG (G) and λ (L) antisera, and is therefore of IgG λ type. (b) Data from lane 23 presented graphically and numerically.

e.g. with high-dose melphalan, followed by autologous peripheral blood stem cell transplant (PBSCT).

• Most patients relapse and median survival is 4–6 years from diagnosis. Relapsed cases may be retreated with initial therapy or with other combinations.

• Radiotherapy is helpful in relieving pain from localized skeletal disease; hemi-body radiotherapy may help to control systemic disease.

• Allogeneic SCT may be curative if applied to selected patients early in the course of the disease.

• Supportive care includes hydration to prevent/treat renal failure, allopurinol to prevent hyperuricaemia, hydration,

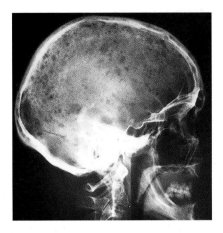

Fig. 24.3 Multiple myeloma: skull X-ray showing multiple lytic lesions.

steroids and bisphosphonates for hypercalcaemia, antibiotics and blood components. Bisphosphonates (e.g. sodium clodronate, pamidronate, zoledronate) are useful in reducing skeletal complications and may improve survival. Surgery may be required for complications (e.g. pathological fracture, spinal cord compression). Plasma exchange is helpful in reducing the paraprotein level quickly.

Related disorders

Benign monoclonal gammopathy (also termed monoclonal gammopathy of undetermined significance, MGUS) is an indolent disorder, more common than myeloma and characterized by a low (<20 g/L) and stationary serum level of paraprotein, no reduction in normal immunoglobulins, absence of skeletal abnormalities and of Bence Jones protein and less than 10% plasma cells in the marrow. It may progress slowly to myeloma or lymphoma in approximately 10–30% of patients.

Primary amyloidosis also shows less than 10% marrow plasma cells and no skeletal lesions but Bence Jones protein and low-level serum paraprotein may occur (see p. 99). Treatment as for myeloma may be beneficial.

Solitary plasmacytoma may occur in bone or in soft tissues, a low level of serum paraprotein may occur and some cases later develop myeloma.

Waldenström's macroglobulinaemia is a chronic lymphoproliferative disorder with a median age at diagnosis of 72 years, and is associated with an IgM paraprotein. Hyperviscosity is common and may cause visual disturbance, central nervous system changes (confusion, impaired conscious level) and headache. Cells resembling plasma cells and lymphocytes are present in the marrow and often in the spleen and lymph nodes.

Plasma cell leukaemia is an aggressive disorder in which large numbers of plasma cells circulate. The prognosis is poor.

25 Lymphoma I: Hodgkin lymphoma (Hodgkin's disease)

Lymphoma is a neoplastic proliferation of lymphoid cells originating in lymph nodes or other lymphoid tissue. It is a heterogeneous group of disorders, divided into Hodgkin lymphoma (HL) and non-Hodgkin lymphoma (NHL). Approximately 200 new cases are diagnosed each year per million population, with a ratio of NHL/HL of approximately 6:1; the incidence is rising.

Aetiology and epidemiology

Hodgkin lymphoma is more prevalent in males than females (M/F ratio 1.5–2.0:1) and has a peak incidence in age range of 15–40 years. The cause is not known, but Epstein–Barr virus (EBV) infection may be a cofactor.

Histological classification

This is well defined and of prognostic significance (see p. 72). Reed–Sternberg (RS) cells are characteristic of HL (Fig. 25.1) and are usually outnumbered by a non-malignant reactive infiltrate of eosinophils, plasma cells, lymphocytes and histiocytes. HL is of B-cell origin.

Clinical features

• Enlarged, painless lymphadenopathy (typically cervical) is the characteristic presentation. The nodes often fluctuate in size, and alcohol ingestion may precipitate pain.
• Hepatic and splenic enlargement may occur.
• Systemic symptoms (fever, weight loss, pruritus and drenching night sweats) occur in 25%.
• Extranodal disease is uncommon but lung, CNS, skin and bone involvement may occur.
• Infection caused by defective cell-mediated/humoral immunity (Fig. 25.3).

Laboratory features

• Anaemia (normochromic, normocytic).
• Leucocytosis (occasionally eosinophilia).
• Leuco-erythroblastic blood film.
• Raised erythrocyte sedimentation rate (ESR), raised lactate dehydrogenase (LDH)—useful as prognostic marker and for monitoring response—and abnormal liver function tests.

Staging

Staging influences both treatment and prognosis. Clinical staging with careful physical examination is followed by cervical thoracic, abdominal and pelvic CT or MRI scanning (Fig. 25.3). Bone marrow aspirate and trephine are performed to detect marrow involvement. The most commonly used staging system is the Cotswold Classification (Fig. 25.4).

Treatment

This depends principally on stage.
• Radiotherapy alone may be used for patients with clinical or pathological stage IA or IIA disease with favourable histology.
• Advanced (stages IB, IIB, III and IV) HD should be treated with combination chemotherapy (CCT) using one of the standard regimes (e.g. six cycles of Adriamycin, bleomycin, vinblastine and dacarbazine, ABVD).
• For bulky mediastinal disease, especially common in young females with nodular sclerosing HL, chemotherapy followed by deep X-ray therapy (DXT) (combined modality therapy) may be given and local DXT may be needed for other sites of bulky or resistant disease.

For complications of treatment see Chapter 39.

Relapsed disease

Patients who relapse following DXT alone generally have a

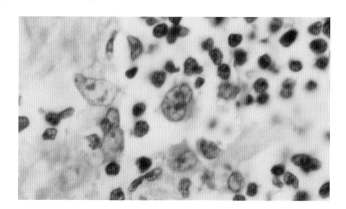

Fig. 25.1 Hodgkin lymphoma: lymph node biopsy showing a Reed–Sternberg cell (multinucleate cell).

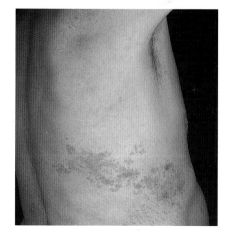

Fig. 25.2 Hodgkin lymphoma: varicella zoster infection.

very good response to CCT (>80% complete remission (CR) rate). Patients initially treated with chemotherapy who relapse after a remission lasting more than 1 year are likely to achieve CR again, and up to 50% may be cured with CCT. However, patients relapsing within 1 year of initial therapy, or failing to achieve complete remission, have a poorer prognosis and should be considered for high-dose therapy with stem cell rescue (see Chapter 38).

Prognosis

Stage is of paramount importance for HL. While >90% of stage I and II may be cured, the rate falls progressively to 50% of stage IV patients. Older patients generally do less well, as do those with lymphocyte-depleted histology.

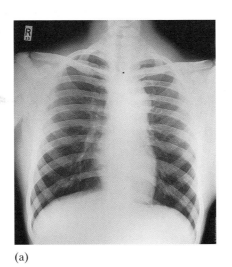 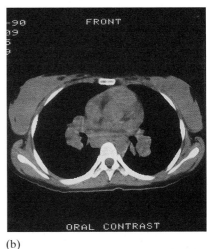

Fig. 25.3 Hodgkin lymphoma: (a) chest X-ray and (b) CT scan showing hilar lymphadenopathy.

(a)   (b)

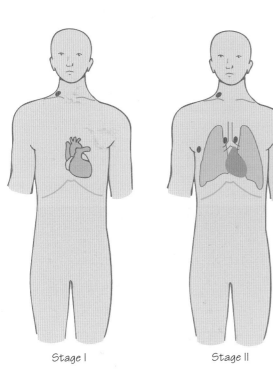 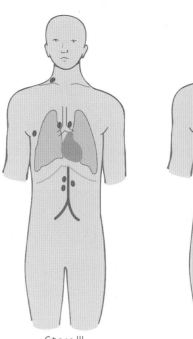 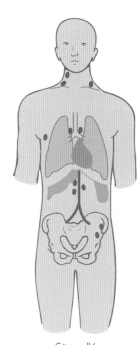

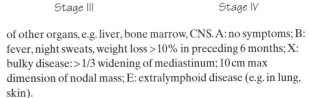

Stage I   Stage II   Stage III   Stage IV

Fig. 25.4 Hodgkin lymphoma: clinical features and staging. Stage I: involvement of a single lymph node region or structure; stage II: involvement of two or more lymph node regions on the same side of the diaphragm; stage III: involvement of lymph node regions or structures on both sides of the diaphragm; stage IV: involvement of other organs, e.g. liver, bone marrow, CNS. A: no symptoms; B: fever, night sweats, weight loss >10% in preceding 6 months; X: bulky disease: >1/3 widening of mediastinum; 10 cm max dimension of nodal mass; E: extralymphoid disease (e.g. in lung, skin).

Lymphoma II: Non-Hodgkin lymphoma

The non-Hodgkin lymphomas (NHLs) are a diverse group of disorders, which encompass a range of clinical presentations, histological appearances and prognostic categories.

Aetiology and epidemiology

Non-Hodgkin lymphoma occurs at all ages, with indolent tumours being most common in the elderly. There is clonal expansion from a normal cell which is 'frozen' at a particular level of differentiation. Most NHLs are B-cell disorders. Environmental factors include abnormal response to viral infection, e.g. Epstein–Barr virus (EBV) in Burkitt's lymphoma (BL) and human T-cell leukaemia virus (HTLV-1) in adult T-cell leukaemia lymphoma (ATLL), or to bacterial infection (e.g. chronic *Helicobacter pylori* infection in gastric lymphoma), or to radiation or certain drugs (e.g. phenytoin). Autoimmune disease (e.g. Sjögren's syndrome, rheumatoid arthritis) and immune suppression (e.g. AIDS, post-transplant) also predispose to NHL. Chromosome translocations in NHL involving oncogenes and immunoglobulin genes include t(14;18) (follicular lymphoma, BCL-2 oncogene) and t(8;14) (BL, MYC oncogene).

Histological classification

At least six different classifications for NHL have existed but NHL is now classified as disease entities based on clinical, biological and histological criteria in the REAL system (see p. 72). Membrane marker and molecular studies of NHL show most (>80%) to be derived from B cells (either follicle centre or from other zones in the lymph node), and the remainder are T cell or unclassified. Indolent NHL may evolve into aggressive disease (Figs 26.1–26.4).

Clinical features
General

• Similar to Hodgkin lymphoma (HL), including painless lymphadenopathy, hepatic and splenic enlargement, systemic symptoms and infection.
• Extranodal disease is more common in NHL than in HL. Thus, gastrointestinal, central nervous system, skin, endocrine organ (including testes), pulmonary and ocular lymphomas will all have the characteristic presenting features of tumours affecting these organs.

Clinical features of sub types of non-Hodgkin lymphoma

Non-Hodgkin lymphoma is clinically heterogeneous, but various clinical patterns emerge.
• Chronic lymphocytic leukaemia (CLL)-like: indolent NHL (small lymphocytic lymphoma (SLL), follicular lymphoma) is more common in older patients (>60 years), is widely disseminated at presentation and may only warrant observation, not treatment. Variants include some T-cell NHL (T-NHL) (e.g. mycosis fungoides) which affect the skin, and splenic marginal zone lymphoma predominantly causing splenomegaly.
• Myeloma-like: bony disease is uncommon but a paraprotein, lymphadenopathy and splenomegaly may occur with lymphoplasmacytoid lymphomas and Waldenström's macroglobulinaemia (see p.67).
• Gastrointestinal lymphomas include mucosa-associated lymphoid tissue (MALT) lymphoma, and T-cell NHL complicating coeliac disease.
• Epidemiology-defined aggressive NHL includes BL (African children, higher incidence in males than females,

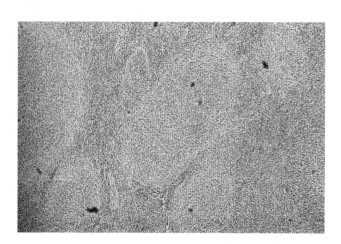

Fig. 26.1 Low-grade (indolent) NHL: lymph node biopsy showing follicular (nodular) structure.

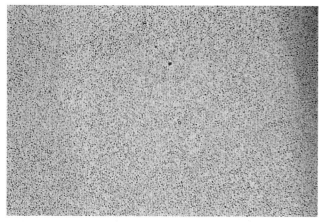

Fig. 26.2 High grade (diffuse) NHL: lymph node biopsy showing diffuse replacement of the node with large cells and destruction of normal nodal architecture.

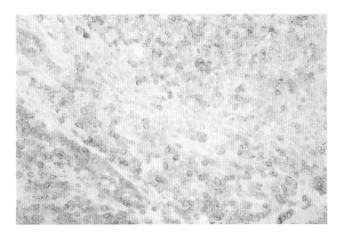

Fig. 26.3 Low-grade NHL: immunostaining showing presence of BCL-2 protein (brown), which prevents apoptosis.

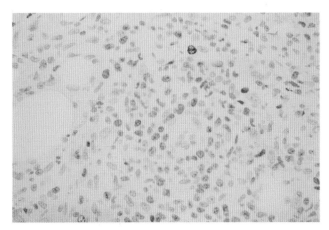

Fig. 26.4 High-grade NHL: immunostaining showing positive staining for Ki67, indicating high proliferation rate.

jaw tumours, EBV related); ATLL (Caribbean and Japan, hypercalcaemia, skin and lymphoid area involvement; HTLV-1 related) and AIDS-related NHL (usually aggressive and frequent central nervous system disease).

Laboratory features
In addition to the changes seen in HL, NHL may cause:
• pancytopenia as a result of bone marrow involvement leading to bone marrow failure;
• peripheral blood lymphocytosis caused by the presence of lymphoma cells in the blood; and
• paraprotein and hypogammaglobulinaemia.

Staging
This is of less importance than in HL. More than 50% of patients with indolent NHL have stage IV disease, whereas aggressive NHL is often of early stage.

Treatment
This depends principally on histology. Paradoxically, aggressive tumours respond more dramatically to treatment and are more likely to be cured than indolent tumours; however, they are also more aggressive if untreated, frequently relapse and are associated with higher short- to medium-term mortality.

Aggressive
Localized (stage I or II) aggressive NHL, deep X-ray therapy (DXT) with adjuvant combination chemotherapy (CCT) (e.g. three cycles of CHOP, a 21-day cycle of cyclophosphamide, hydroxydaunorubicin (Adriamycin), vincristine and prednisolone). Advanced stage aggressive NHL is treated with CCT (up to complete remission plus at least two cycles) followed by DXT to sites of bulky disease. Patients with lymphoblastic lymphoma are best treated with the very aggressive CCT regimes used for acute lymphoblastic leukaemia; such patients are candidates for allogeneic stem cell transplantation (see Chapter 38).

Indolent
Asymptomatic patients may be followed closely without therapy for months or even years. When treatment is required, options include DXT, single agent chemotherapy (e.g. oral chlorambucil) and CCT with or without DXT. The relapse rate is high. Trials of aggressive chemotherapy followed by stem cell transplantation are in progress for younger patients.

Relapsed disease
Over 50% of NHL patients will relapse after initial therapy. Indolent NHL will typically respond to single agent, CCT or radiotherapy. Relapsed aggressive NHL carries a poor prognosis but may respond to second-line CCT regimes followed by autologous or allogeneic stem cell transplantation.

New therapies
The use of monoclonal antibodies, interleukin-2, interferon, new chemotherapeutic agents (e.g. fludarabine, 2-chlorodeoxy-adenosine (2-CDA) in indolent lymphomas) and the use of antisense oligonucleotides to the oncogene BCL-2 are under current investigation.

Prognosis
Prognosis in NHL is largely dependent on histology. The presence of bulky disease, multiple sites of extranodal involvement, age, performance status and laboratory parameters, such as LDH level and $\beta2$ microglobulin level, all influence prognosis. Long-term side effects of therapy are considered in Chapter 39.

The REAL classification

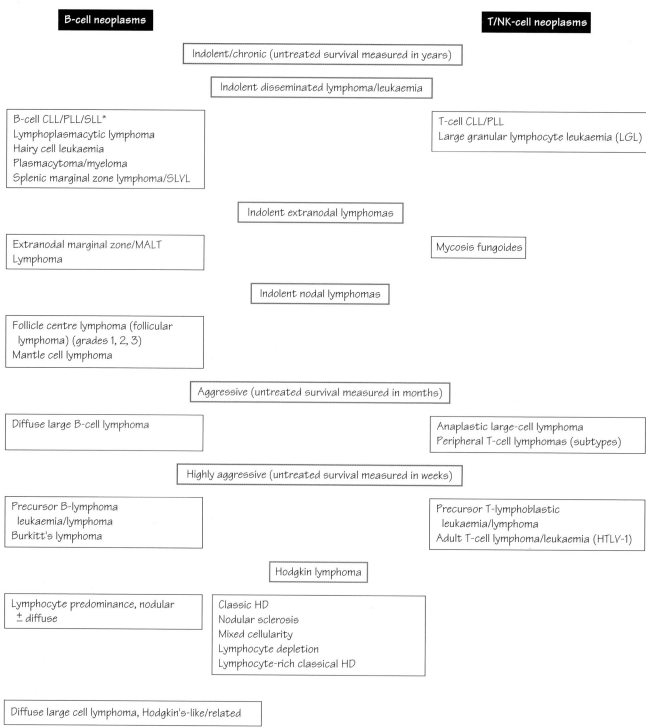

B-cell neoplasms

T/NK-cell neoplasms

Indolent/chronic (untreated survival measured in years)

Indolent disseminated lymphoma/leukaemia

B-cell CLL/PLL/SLL*
Lymphoplasmacytic lymphoma
Hairy cell leukaemia
Plasmacytoma/myeloma
Splenic marginal zone lymphoma/SLVL

T-cell CLL/PLL
Large granular lymphocyte leukaemia (LGL)

Indolent extranodal lymphomas

Extranodal marginal zone/MALT
Lymphoma

Mycosis fungoides

Indolent nodal lymphomas

Follicle centre lymphoma (follicular
lymphoma) (grades 1, 2, 3)
Mantle cell lymphoma

Aggressive (untreated survival measured in months)

Diffuse large B-cell lymphoma

Anaplastic large-cell lymphoma
Peripheral T-cell lymphomas (subtypes)

Highly aggressive (untreated survival measured in weeks)

Precursor B-lymphoma
leukaemia/lymphoma
Burkitt's lymphoma

Precursor T-lymphoblastic
leukaemia/lymphoma
Adult T-cell lymphoma/leukaemia (HTLV-1)

Hodgkin lymphoma

Lymphocyte predominance, nodular
± diffuse

Classic HD
Nodular sclerosis
Mixed cellularity
Lymphocyte depletion
Lymphocyte-rich classical HD

Diffuse large cell lymphoma, Hodgkin's-like/related

* Small lymphocytic lymphoma

The REAL (Revised European American Lymphoma) classification. CLL, chronic lymphocytic leukaemia; HD, Hodgkin's disease; PLL, prolymphocytic leukaemia; SLL, small lymphocytic lymphoma; SLVL, splenic lymphoma with villous lymphocytes.

27 Myeloproliferative disorders

Myeloproliferative disorders (MPD) are chronic diseases caused by clonal proliferation of bone marrow stem cells leading to excess production of one or more haemopoietic lineage (Fig. 27.1). The clinical syndromes include poly-cythaemia rubra vera (red cells), essential thrombo-cythaemia (platelets), chronic myeloid leukaemia (white cells) and myelofibrosis in which there is a reactive fibrosis of the marrow and extramedullary haemopoiesis in the liver and spleen. Intermediate forms may occur and the diseases may all transform into acute myeloid leukaemia. Their combined overall incidence is 100–150 cases/year/ million population in Europe.

Polycythaemia

Polycythaemia (erythrocytosis) is defined as an increase in haemoglobin concentration above normal (Table 27.1). True polycythaemia exists when the total red cell mass (RCM), measured by dilution of isotopically labelled red cells, is increased above normal. Spurious (pseudo or stress) polycythaemia exists when an elevated haemoglobin concentration is caused by a reduction in plasma volume, measured by dilution of isotopically labelled albumin.

Polycythaemia rubra vera
Aetiology and pathophysiology
Polycythaemia rubra vera (PRV) is a primary neo-

Table 27.1 Causes of polycythaemia.

True polycythaemia

Primary
Polycythaemia rubra vera (PRV)

Secondary
Erythropoietin appropriately increased
  High altitude
  Cyanotic congenital heart disease
  Chronic lung disease
  Haemoglobin variant with increased oxygen affinity
Erythropoietin inappropriately increased
  Renal disease: hypernephroma, renal cyst, hydronephrosis
  Uterine myoma
  Other tumours, e.g. hepatocellular carcinoma, bronchial
    carcinoma

Relative (spurious) polycythaemia

Plasma volume depletion
Stress ('pseudo-polycythaemia')
Dehydration
Diuretic therapy

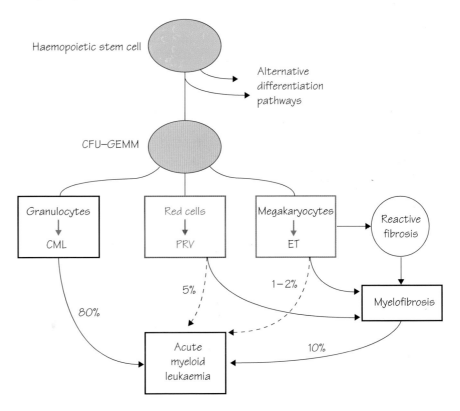

Fig. 27.1 The myeloproliferative disorders.

plastic disorder in which bone marrow erythropoiesis is increased, usually accompanied by increased thrombopoiesis and granulopoiesis. Serum erythropoietin (EPO) levels are low.

Clinical features
- Polycythaemia rubra vera occurs equally in males and females, typically over 55 years of age.
- Raised RCM causes a ruddy complexion (Fig. 27.2) and conjunctival suffusion; hyperviscosity may lead to headaches and visual disturbance.
- Thrombosis (e.g. deep vein thrombosis (DVT), Budd–Chiari syndrome, stroke) are also caused by hyperviscosity and increased platelets.
- Haemorrhage, especially gastrointestinal, may occur.
- Excess histamine secretion from basophils leads to increased gastric acid and peptic ulcer is frequent.
- Pruritus, typically after a hot bath, and gout, caused by increased uric acid production, also occur frequently.
- Enlarged spleen is found in 75% of patients and distinguishes PRV from other causes of polycythaemia (Fig. 27.3).

Laboratory features
- Raised haematocrit, haemoglobin concentration, red cell count and RCM.
- Seventy-five per cent of all patients have raised white cells (neutrophil leucocytosis) and/or platelets.
- Neutrophil alkaline phosphatase (NAP) score, serum B_{12}, serum B_{12} binding capacity and serum uric acid are all usually raised.
- Bone marrow is hypercellular with prominent megakaryocytes, iron stores are depleted because of excessive iron

utilization, and the trephine biopsy may show mildly increased reticulin.
- Abdominal ultrasound excludes renal disease and assesses spleen size.
- Culture of peripheral blood cells shows spontaneous formation of erythroid colonies.

Differential diagnosis
Secondary or reactive polycythaemia may occur in conditions where arterial oxygen saturation is reduced, leading to a physiological rise in EPO, or when EPO levels are inappropriately raised (e.g. caused by secretion of EPO by a renal neoplasm).

Spurious (*pseudo*) *polycythaemia* arises when plasma volume is reduced by dehydration, vomiting or diuretic therapy. A common form occurs particularly in young male adults, especially smokers, and is associated with stress, increased vasomotor tone and hypertension (Gaisböck's syndrome). The white cell and platelet counts are normal, as is the bone marrow and RCM. If the packed cell volume (PCV) is over 0.50, it is treated by venesections; patients should reduce weight, stop smoking, moderate alcohol intake and avoid diuretics.

The following additional tests are occasionally required.
- Chest X-ray; arterial blood gas analysis to exclude lung disease.
- Haemoglobin oxygen dissociation curve to identify a variant haemoglobin with increased oxygen affinity.
- Serum EPO assay.

Treatment
- Thrombosis is the main cause of morbidity and mortality and its incidence can be reduced by maintaining the PCV below 0.45 and platelets below 600×10^9/L. Aspirin (75 mg daily) is often used to inhibit platelet function.
- Regular venesection is used initially to lower the PCV.
- Chemotherapy (e.g. oral hydroxyurea) is also usually required.
- ^{32}P is a β-emitter which is taken up and concentrated by bone and may be used to give prolonged myelosuppression (about 2 years) in older patients.

Prognosis
Median survival is about 16 years. Up to 30% of patients develop myelofibrosis (see below). Acute myeloid leukaemia occurs in up to 5% of patients, probably increased in patients treated with a ^{32}P and some types of chemotherapy.

Essential thrombocythaemia
Essential thrombocythaenia (ET) is defined as persistent elevation of the peripheral blood platelet count as a result of increased marrow production in the absence of a systemic cause for thrombocytosis (Table 27.2).

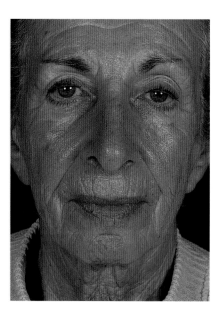

Fig. 27.2 Polycythaemia rubra vera patient with plethora.

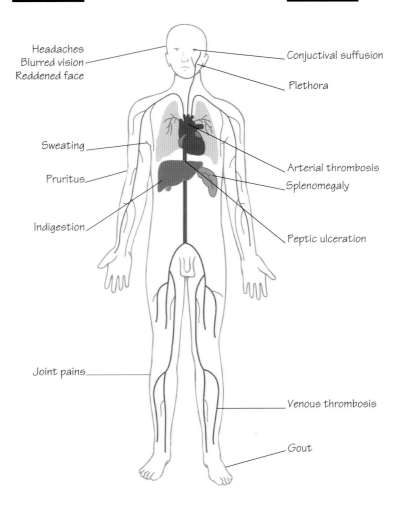

Headaches
Blurred vision
Reddened face

Conjuctival suffusion

Plethora

Sweating

Pruritus

Arterial thrombosis

Splenomegaly

Indigestion

Peptic ulceration

Joint pains

Venous thrombosis

Gout

Fig. 27.3 Polycythaemia rubra vera: clinical features.

Table 27.2 Causes of an elevated platelet count.

Primary

Essential thrombocythaemia
As part of another myeloproliferative disorder, e.g. PRV, CML,
   myelofibrosis

Reactive

Iron deficiency
Haemorrhage
Severe haemolysis
Trauma, postoperatively
Infection, inflammation
Malignancy
Hyposplenism

CML, chronic myeloid leukaemia; PRV, polycythaemia rubra
vera.

Aetiology and pathophysiology
Similar to PRV, distinction between the two conditions is
not exact. ET occurs more frequently in younger adults
than PRV.

Clinical features
• Thrombosis, both arterial (peripheral vessels with gan-
grene of toes, cerebral, coronary and mesenteric ar-
teries) and venous (e.g. Budd–Chiari syndrome, DVT).
Headaches, visual disturbance and peripheral vascular
disease occur.
• At least 20% of patients are asymptomatic and detected
as an incidental finding.
• Excessive haemorrhage may occur spontaneously or
after trauma or surgery.
• Pruritus and sweating are uncommon.
• Splenomegaly in about 30% of patients; in others the
spleen is atrophied because of infarction.

Laboratory features

- Platelet count is persistently raised and often >1000× 10^9/L, raised red cell and/or white cell count is present in about 30% (Fig. 27.4).
- Blood film shows platelet anisocytosis with circulating megakaryocyte fragments. Autoinfarction of the spleen causes changes in red cells (target cells, Howell–Jolly bodies).
- The NAP score may be raised or normal.
- Serum uric acid is often raised, serum LDH may be raised.
- Bone marrow is hypercellular with increased numbers of megakaryocytes, often in aggregates.
- Defective platelet function, especially defective aggregation in response to adenosine diphosphate (ADP) and adrenaline, may help to distinguish primary from reactive thrombocythaemia.

Treatment

- Chemotherapy, e.g. hydroxyurea, is used to maintain the platelet count below 600× 10^9/L.
- α-Interferon and oral anagrelide are also effective.
- Aspirin (75 mg daily), except in those with haemorrhage.

Prognosis

Median survival is more than 20 years; thrombosis and haemorrhage are the main causes of morbidity and mortality. Transformation to AML may occur.

Myelofibrosis

Myelofibrosis (myelosclerosis, agnogenic myeloid metaplasia) is characterized by splenomegaly, extramedullary haemopoiesis, a leuco-erythroblastic blood picture and replacement of bone marrow by collagen fibrosis.

Aetiology and pathophysiology

Primary defect is within the haemopoietic stem cell; fibrosis results from a reactive non-neoplastic proliferation of marrow stromal cells. One-third of patients have a preceding history of PRV or essential thrombocythaemia.

Clinical features

- Sexes affected equally; age of onset rarely below 50 years.
- Massive splenomegaly may lead to left hypochondrial pain and anaemia, leucopenia and thrombocytopenia (hypersplenism) (Fig. 27.5).
- Fever, weight loss, pruritus, hepatomegaly and night sweats are frequent; gout, bone and joint pain are less common.
- Abdominal swelling, ascites and bleeding from oesophageal varices occur, caused by portal hypertension, in late stages.

Laboratory features

- Normochromic normocytic anaemia.
- Leucocytosis and thrombocytosis with circulating megakaryocyte fragments occur early; leucopenia and thrombocytopenia later.
- Blood film: red cell poikilocytosis with teardrop forms and circulating red cell and white cell precursors (leuco-erythroblastic picture) (Fig. 27.6).
- Serum LDH is raised. Liver function tests are often abnormal because of extramedullary haemopoiesis.
- NAP score, serum B_{12} and B_{12} binding capacity are usually raised.
- Bone marrow aspiration is usually unsuccessful ('dry tap'); the trephine biopsy shows increased cellularity, increased megakaryocytes and fibrosis (Figs 27.7 and 27.8).

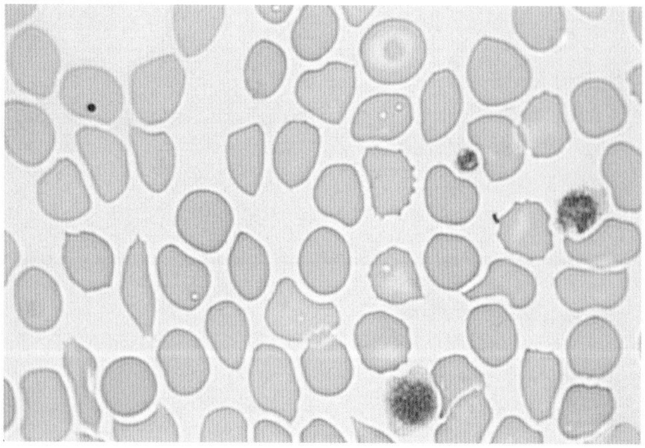

Fig. 27.4 Essential thrombocythaemia: peripheral blood film showing increased numbers of platelets, giant platelets and changes of hyposplenism because of splenic autoinfarction.

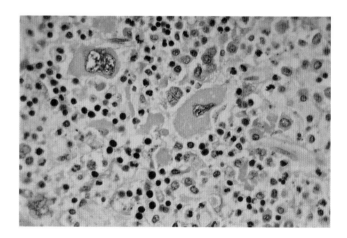

Fig. 27.5 Myelofibrosis: spleen section showing extramedullary haemopoiesis.

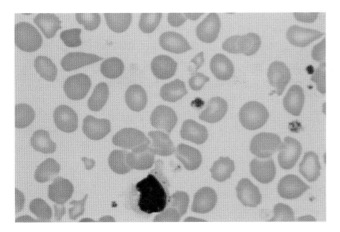

Fig. 27.6 Myelofibrosis: peripheral blood film showing aniso/poikilocytosis, teardrop forms and giant platelets.

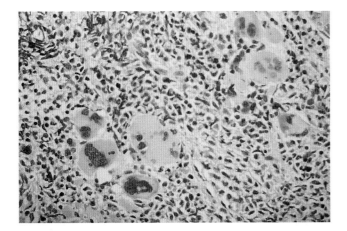

Fig. 27.7 Myelofibrosis: bone marrow biopsy showing increased cellularity and large numbers of megakaryocytes.

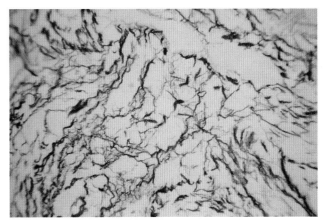

Fig. 27.8 Myelofibrosis: bone marrow biopsy (reticulin stain) showing increased reticulin.

Treatment

• Chemotherapy (e.g. hydroxyurea) for patients with hypermetabolism and myeloproliferation.
• Supportive therapy with red cell transfusions, folic acid and occasionally platelet transfusions. Iron chelation may be needed.
• Allopurinol to prevent hyperuricaemia and gout.
• Splenectomy or splenic irradiation to reduce symptoms from splenomegaly, anaemia or thrombocytopenia (selected patients only).
• Allogeneic bone marrow transplantation has cured a few younger patients (<50 years).

Prognosis

Median survival is about 5 years; acute leukaemia occurs in about 20%.

Haemostasis (Fig. 28.1) is the process whereby haemorrhage following vascular injury is arrested. It depends on closely linked interaction between:
• the vessel wall;
• platelets; and
• coagulation factors.

The fibrinolytic system and inhibitors of coagulation ensure coagulation is limited to the site of injury.

The vessel wall

The intact vessel wall has an important role in preventing haemostasis. Endothelial cells produce:
• prostacyclin, which causes vasodilatation and inhibits platelet aggregation;
• Protein C (PC) activator (thrombomodulin), which inhibits coagulation; and
• tissue plasminogen activator (TPA) which activates fibrinolysis.

Injury to the vessel wall: (i) activates membrane bound tissue factor which initiates coagulation (Fig. 28.2); and (ii) exposes subendothelial connective tissue allowing binding of platelets to von Willebrand factor (vWF), a large, multimeric protein made by endothelial cells, which mediates platelet adhesion to endothelium and carries clotting factor VIII in plasma.

Platelets (see Chapter 2)

Platelets have a large surface area onto which coagulation factors are absorbed. Glycoproteins GPIb and IIb/IIIa allow attachment of platelets to vWF (Fig. 28.3) and hence to endothelium. Collagen exposure and thrombin promote platelet aggregation and the platelet release reaction whereby platelets release their granule contents. Adenosine diphosphate (ADP) promotes platelet aggregation to form a primary haemostatic plug. Platelet prostaglandin synthesis is activated to form thromboxane A_2 which poten-

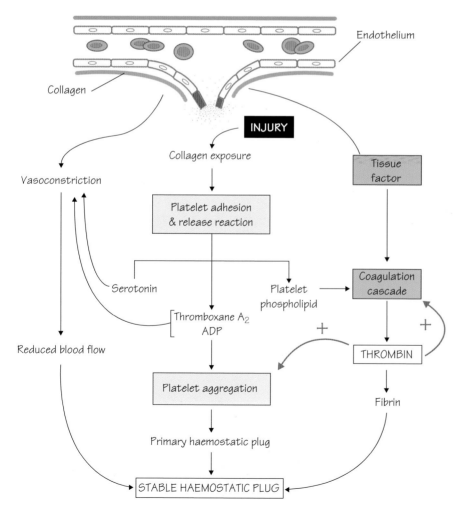

Fig. 28.1 Haemostasis.

tiates the platelet release reaction, promotes platelet aggregation and also has vasoconstrictor activity. Fibrin, produced by blood coagulation, binds to vWF and enmeshes the platelets to form a stable haemostatic plug. Activated platelets promote coagulation, as they have exposed phospholipid binding sites (the prothrombinase complex) which are involved in activation of factor X and of prothrombin to thrombin in the coagulation cascade.

Coagulation factors

The proteins of the coagulation cascade are proenzymes (serine proteases) and procofactors which are activated sequentially (Fig. 28.2). The cascade has been divided on the basis of laboratory tests into intrinsic, extrinsic and common pathways. This division is useful in understanding results of *in vitro* coagulation tests. *In vivo*, however, these pathways are closely interlinked. Coagulation begins when tissue factor activated on the surface of injured cells binds and activates factor VII; the complex activates factor IX which, with cofactor VIII, activates factor X to Xa.

Platelets accelerate the coagulation process by providing membrane phospholipid. The complex of Xa and Va, activated from cofactor V by thrombin, acts on prothrombin (factor II) to generate thrombin. Thrombin then converts fibrinogen into fibrin monomers, with release of fibrinopeptides A and B. The monomers combine to form a fibrin

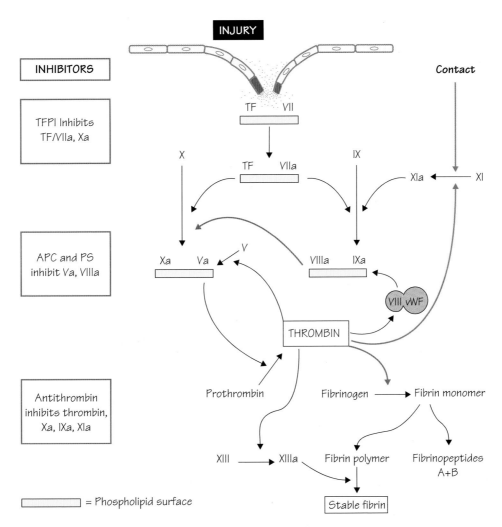

Fig. 28.2 The coagulation pathway. Injury initiates release of tissue factor (TF). Tissue factor binds and activates factor VII. The TF VIIa complex activates factors X and IX; the activity of the TF VIIa complex is inhibited by TF pathway inhibitor (TFPI). The VIIIa–IXa complex amplifies Xa production from X. Thrombin is generated from prothrombin by the action of Xa–Va complex and this leads to fibrin formation. Thrombin also: (i) activates FXI leading to increased FIXa production; (ii) cleaves FVIII from its carrier protein vWF activating FVIII; (iii) activates FV to FVa; and (iv) activates FXIII to XIIIa, which stabilizes the fibrin clot. Note that: (i) TFPI inhibits TF/VIIa, Xa; (ii) Activated PC (APC) and PS inhibit Va, VIIIa; and (iii) antithrombin inhibits thrombin, Xa, IXa. Extrinsic pathway, Factor VII. Intrinsic pathway, Factors XI, IX, VIII. Common pathway, Factors X, V, II, fibrinogen.

polymer clot. Factor XIII crosslinks the polymer to form a more stable clot.

Thrombin has a number of key roles in the coagulation process.

1 It converts plasma fibrinogen into fibrin.

2 It amplifies coagulation by: (i) activating factor XI which increases IXa production; (ii) cleaving factor VIII from its carrier molecule vWF to activate it and augment Xa production; and (iii) activating factor V to factor Va.

3 It activates factor XIII to factor XIIIa, which stabilizes the fibrin clot.

4 It potentiates platelet aggregation.

5 It binds to thrombomodulin on the endothelial cell surface to form a complex which activates protein C, which is involved in regulating coagulation.

Coagulation inhibitory factors

These inhibit the coagulation cascade and ensure the action of thrombin is limited to the site of injury.

1 Antithrombin inactivates serine proteases, principally factor Xa and thrombin. Heparin activates antithrombin.

2 α_2 Macroglobulins, α_2 antiplasmin, α_2 antitrypsin and heparin cofactor II also inhibit circulating serine proteases.

3 Proteins C and S are vitamin K-dependent proteins made in the liver. Protein C is activated via a thrombin–thrombomodulin complex (Fig. 32.2) and, like protein S, inhibits coagulation by inactivating factors Va and VIIIa; it also enhances fibrinolysis by inactivating the tissue plasmogen activator (TPA) inhibitor (see Fig. 28.4).

4 Tissue factor pathway inhibitor (TFPI) inhibits the main *in vivo* coagulation pathway by inhibiting factor VIIa and Xa.

The fibrinolytic pathway (Fig. 28.4)

Fibrinolysis is the process whereby fibrin is degraded by plasmin. A circulating pro-enzyme, plasminogen, may be activated to plasmin:

1 following injury, by TPA and urokinase-like plasminogen activator (UPA) released from damaged or activated cells; or

2 by exogenous agents, e.g. streptokinase, or by therapeutic TPA or UPA.

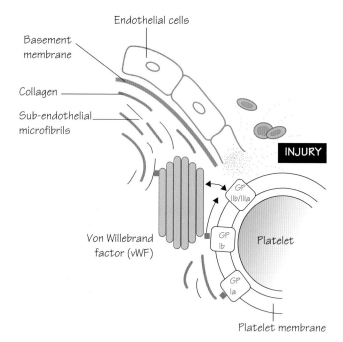

Fig. 28.3 Platelet adhesion. Subendothelial microfibrils bind von Willebrand factor (vWF) which in turn binds platelets at the glycoprotein 1b (GP1b) receptor. This binding exposes the platelet glycoprotein IIb/IIIa (GPIIb/IIIa) receptor which binds further with vWF. The GPIIb/IIIa receptor also binds fibrinogen to allow platelet–platelet aggregation. The platelet glycoprotein 1a (GP1a) receptor binds directly to collagen.

Table 28.1 Laboratory tests of coagulation.

Screening test (normal range)	Abnormalities indicated (prolonged abnormal)	Most common cause of disorder
Prothrombin time (PT) (10–14s)	Extrinsic and common coagulation pathways Deficiency/inhibition of factor VII, factors X, V, II and fibrinogen	Liver disease, Warfarin therapy, DIC
Activated partial thromblastin time (APTT or PTTK) (30–40s)	Intrinsic and common coagulation pathways Deficiency/inhibition of one or more of factors XII, IX, VIII, X, V, II and fibrinogen	Liver disease, heparin therapy, haemophilia A and B, DIC
Thrombin time (14–16s)	Deficiency or abnormality of fibrinogen; inhibition of thrombin by heparin or FDPs	DIC, heparin therapy, fibrinolytic therapy
Fibrin degradation products (<10mg/mL)	Accelerated destruction of fibrinogen	DIC
Bleeding time (5–8min)	Abnormal platelet function	Drugs (e.g. aspirin), uraemia, von Willebrand's disease
Euglobulin clot lysis time	Fibrinolytic pathway defect	Smoking

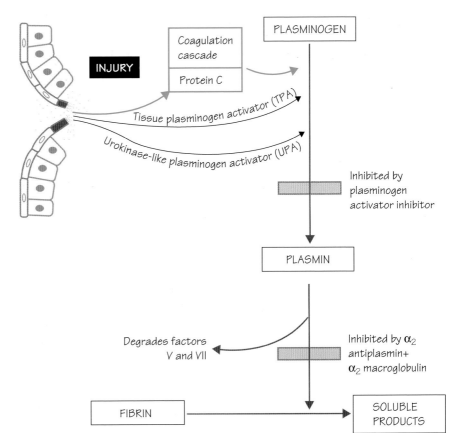

Fig. 28.4 Fibrinolysis. Injury causes release of TPA and UPA which, together with activated components from coagulation pathway and protein C, activate plasminogen to plasmin. Plasmin acts on insoluble fibrin to form a series of soluble products (fragment X, fragments Y + D, fragments E + D). Note that: (i) plasminogen activator inhibitor inhibits activation of plasminogen; and (ii) α_2 antiplasmin and α_2 macroglobulin inhibit action of plasmin.

Plasmin digests fibrin (or fibrinogen) into fibrin degradation products (FDPs) and also degrades factors V and VII. Free plasmin is inactivated by plasma α_2 antiplasmin and α_2 macroglobulin.

Laboratory tests of coagulation
These are listed in Table 28.1.

Specialized tests
Individual coagulation factors can be assayed by functional tests or immunological methods. Platelet function tests include tests of platelet aggregation with different agonists, platelet adhesion and assessment of platelet granule contents. Tests for abnormalities leading to thrombosis (thrombophilia) are described in Chapter 32.

29 Disorders of haemostasis: vessel wall and platelets

Defective haemostasis with abnormal bleeding may be caused by:
- abnormalities of the vessel wall;
- thrombocytopenia;
- disordered platelet function; and
- defective blood coagulation (see Chapters 30 and 31).

Vessel wall abnormalities
These are associated with easy bruising, purpura and ecchymosis and spontaneous bleeding from mucosal surfaces. The bleeding time, prothrombin time (PT), activated partial thromboplastin time (APTT) and platelet count are all normal.

Inherited
- Hereditary haemorrhagic telangiectasia. This is autosomal dominant with multiple dilated microvascular swellings, typically in oropharynx (Fig. 29.1) and gastrointestinal tract, which bleed spontaneously or following minor trauma. Local treatment (e.g. nasal packing) may control bleeding; tranexamic acid helps to reduce bleeding. Chronic iron deficiency is frequent.
- Ehlers–Danlos syndrome, Marfan's syndrome and other rare connective tissue disorders.

Acquired
Causes include vitamin C deficiency (scurvy), steroid

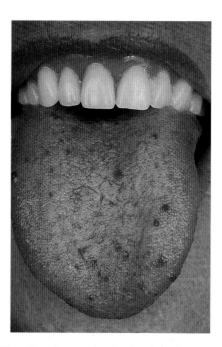

Fig. 29.1 Hereditary haemorrhagic telangiectasia: tongue showing multiple telangiectasia.

therapy, normal ageing (senile purpura) and immune complex deposition (e.g. purpura fulminans in septicaemia). Henoch–Schönlein purpura is an allergic vasculitis which follows an acute infection, usually in childhood, and may be associated with arthropathy, haematuria and gastrointestinal symptoms.

Platelets
Excessive bleeding caused by thrombocytopenia or disordered platelet function is mucosal (e.g. epistaxis, gastrointestinal bleeding or menorrhagia) or affects the skin (purpura, petechiae and ecchymoses). Symptoms usually occur when the platelet count is $<10\times10^9$/L but this may be higher when there is impaired platelet function.

Thrombocytopenia (platelets $<140\times10^9$/L) (Fig. 29.2)
Congenital
This is rare: causes include congenital aplastic anaemia, thrombocytopenia with absent radii (TAR) syndrome or Wiskott–Aldrich syndrome (thrombocytopenia with eczema and hypogammaglobulinaemia). Congenital infection (e.g. rubella, cytomegalovirus) frequently leads to thrombocytopenia.

Acquired
This is a result of deficient platelet production or accelerated platelet destruction.

Immune thrombocytopenia
The platelets are coated with autoantibody (immunoglobulin) and are removed by the macrophages of the reticuloendothelial system. Their lifespan is therefore reduced from 7–10 days to a few hours.

Autoimmune thrombocytopenia
Acute
- Usually presents in childhood (2–7 years).
- Often follows a viral infection.
- Purpuric rash or epistaxis frequent (Figs 29.3 and 29.4).
- Typically resolves spontaneously. A minority develop mucosal bleeding and should be treated with prednisolone or intravenous immunoglobulin. Up to 20% develop chronic immune thrombocytopenia.

Chronic
Immune thrombocytopenia in adults is less likely to resolve without therapy and usually chronic. It is more common in females (M/F ratio 1:4). Autoantibody is present on the platelet surface and may also be present as free antibody in serum.

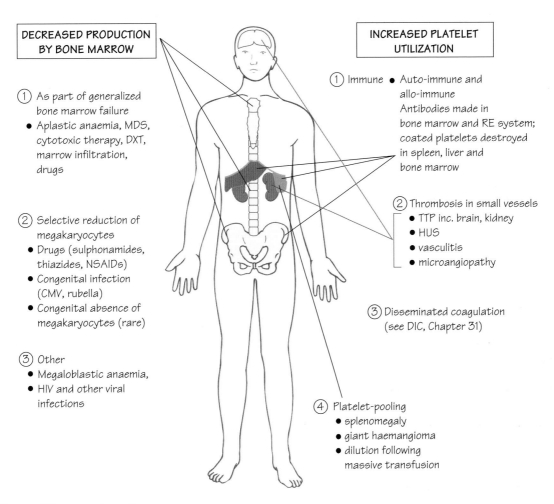

DECREASED PRODUCTION BY BONE MARROW

① As part of generalized bone marrow failure
● Aplastic anaemia, MDS, cytotoxic therapy, DXT, marrow infiltration, drugs

② Selective reduction of megakaryocytes
● Drugs (sulphonamides, thiazides, NSAIDs)
● Congenital infection (CMV, rubella)
● Congenital absence of megakaryocytes (rare)

③ Other
● Megaloblastic anaemia,
● HIV and other viral infections

INCREASED PLATELET UTILIZATION

① Immune ● Auto-immune and allo-immune Antibodies made in bone marrow and RE system; coated platelets destroyed in spleen, liver and bone marrow

② Thrombosis in small vessels
● TTP inc. brain, kidney
● HUS
● vasculitis
● microangiopathy

③ Disseminated coagulation (see DIC, Chapter 31)

④ Platelet-pooling
● splenomegaly
● giant haemangioma
● dilution following massive transfusion

Fig. 29.2 Causes of thrombocytopenia.

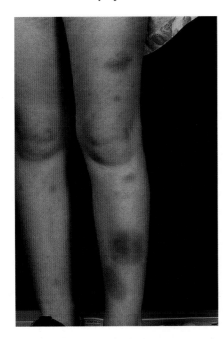

Fig. 29.3 Immune thrombocytopenia: multiple bruises, ecchymoses and purpura.

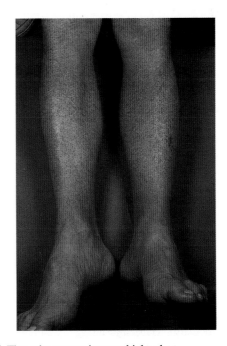

Fig. 29.4 Thrombocytopenia: petechial rash.

Laboratory findings
- Normal haemoglobin and white cell count; platelets low, often $<20\times10^9$/L.
- Bone marrow is normal or increased numbers of megakaryocytes.
- PT and APTT are normal, fibrinogen is normal.

Immune thrombocytopenia also occurs in association with some malignancies (e.g. chronic lymphocytic leukaemia, non-Hodgkin lymphoma, myelodysplasia), infections (e.g. Epstein–Barr virus, HIV, malaria) and connective tissue disease (e.g. systemic lupus erythematosus). Patients should be tested for ANF and anticardiolipin antibodies.

Treatment
Treatment, if necessary, is with the following.
- Prednisolone (1 mg/kg/day, reducing over 4–6 weeks).
- Intravenous immunoglobulin is valuable for obtaining a temporary rise in platelet count.
- Splenectomy is required for non-responders with continuing symptoms and/or very low platelet counts.
- Additional immunosuppressive therapy (e.g. azathioprine, cyclophosphamide, cyclosporin A, rhesus anti-D, vincristine) or even combination chemotherapy have been used.

Alloimmune thrombocytopenia

Transplacental passage of maternal antibody in immune thrombocytopenia can lead to neonatal thrombocytopenia, which typically resolves spontaneously over a few weeks. Mothers who have been sensitized (e.g. by blood transfusion or previous pregnancy) to platelet antigens may develop antibodies which cross the placenta and coat fetal and neonatal platelets, which are then removed in the reticuloendothelial system. Individuals with such platelet alloantibodies can also become thrombocytopenic after blood transfusion (post-transfusion purpura). The antibody usually is directed against the HPA1-a antigen on platelets.

Other causes of thrombocytopenia
Drugs
Drugs cause thrombocytopenia by inhibiting marrow production or by an immune mechanism. The most common immune mechanism (e.g. quinine, heparin) is when the drug forms an antigen with a plasma protein, an antibody is formed to it, and circulating antigen–antibody complexes are absorbed on the platelet surface. Heparin-induced thrombocytopenia is associated with thrombosis.

Disseminated intravascular coagulation
This is discussed in Chapter 31.

Thrombotic thrombocytopenic purpura and haemolytic uraemic syndrome
Thrombotic thrombocytopenic purpura (TTP) and haemolytic uraemic syndrome (HUS) are characterized by thrombosis in small vessels, red cell fragmentation, haemolytic anaemia (Fig. 29.5) and thrombocytopenia. Renal failure often occurs in HUS and fever, neurological changes and liver dysfunction in TTP. The PT and APTT are normal. TTP is caused by a deficiency—either congenital or acquired from an antibody—of a plasma protease which normally cleaves von Willebrand factor (vWF). Abnormally high molecular weight vWF complexes are present in plasma. Haemolytic uraemic syndrome occurs in childhood and follows infection with verotoxin-producing strains of *E. coli*; it is also associated with *Shigella*, *Salmonella* and streptococcal infection, pregnancy, autoimmune diseases and drugs (e.g. cyclosporin A). The protease levels are normal. TTP is more frequently fatal, occurs in adults

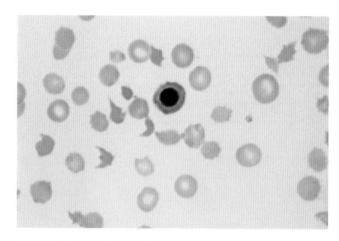

Fig. 29.5 Haemolytic uraemic syndrome: blood film showing red cell fragmentation with a circulating nucleated red blood cell and low platelet count.

Table 29.1 Disorders of platelet function.

Inherited

Bernard–Soulier syndrome (defective glycoprotein 1b, giant platelets)
Glanzmann's thrombasthaenia (defective glycoproteins IIb, IIIa)
Storage pool diseases, von Willebrand's disease (see Chapter 30)

Acquired

Drugs: aspirin, other non-steroidal anti-inflammatory agents, clopidrogel, clopidrogel dextran, antibiotic therapy (e.g. cephalosporins)
Myeloproliferative disorders: polycythaemia rubra vera, essential thrombocythaemia, myelofibrosis
Uraemia
Paraproteinaemia, e.g. myeloma or Waldenström's macroglobulinaemia

and may be associated with autoimmune conditions (e.g. SLE), pregnancy and infection.

Treatment of TTP is with plasma exchange using fresh frozen plasma (FFP) as the replacement fluid. Fresh frozen plasma depleted of cryoprecipitate may be more effective, while FFP which has been solvent treated is less likely to transmit viral infection. Antiplatelet drugs (aspirin or dipyridamole), corticosteroids, splenectomy and vincristine have all been used. Response to treatment may be monitored by haemoglobin level, reticulocytes, lactate dehydrogenase, platelet count, plasma bilirubin and presence of vWF multimers in plasma. In HUS, treatment for fits, hypertension and renal failure may be needed.

Disorders of platelet function (Table 29.1)

These are characterized by a prolonged bleeding time with normal platelet count and disordered platelet aggregation. **Inherited disorders** are rare and present with bruising/excessive bleeding after surgery or injury in childhood. The most common **acquired** cause is aspirin and other non-steroidal anti-inflammatory drugs.

30 Disorders of coagulation I: Inherited

Excessive bleeding may occur as a result of an inherited defect of one or other protein involved in coagulation. Inherited deficiency of each of the coagulation factors has been described. The defects are point mutations, deletions or intragenic inversions.

Factor VIII deficiency (haemophilia A)

Factor VIII deficiency (haemophilia A) is the most common inherited disorder (approximately 50 cases/million population). The factor VIII gene is on the X chromosome so inheritance is sex-linked (Fig. 30.1). A wide range of genetic changes is described including deletions, insertions and point mutations and a common intragene inversion.

Clinical features

- Range from severe spontaneous bleeding, especially into joints (haemarthroses) and muscles, to mild symptoms (Fig. 30.2).
- Onset in early childhood (e.g. postcircumcision).
- Increased risk of postoperative or post-traumatic haemorrhage.
- Chronic debilitating joint disease caused by repeated bleeds.

Laboratory features (Table 30.1)

- Prolonged activated partial thromboplastin time (APTT), normal prothrombin time (PT), normal bleeding time, plasma factor VIII reduced (<1% of normal in severe cases, but up to 10% in mild cases).
- Carriers have factor VIII approximately 50% of normal. DNA analysis is helpful in carrier detection and counselling.
- Von Willebrand factor level is normal.

Treatment (see also Chapter 37)

- Infusions of factor VIII concentrate to elevate the patient's level to 20–50% of normal for severe bleeding.
- Level is raised to and maintained at 80–100% for elective surgery.
- Desmopressin, an analogue of vasopressin, leads to a modest rise in endogenous factor VIII which is useful in mild cases.
- Avoid aspirin, other antiplatelet drugs and intramuscular injections.
- Patients should be registered with a recognized haemophilia centre and should carry a card with details of their condition.
- Patients may need to have continuing or prophylactic treatment at home.

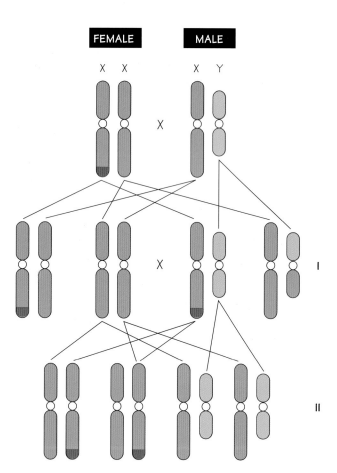

Fig. 30.1 Inheritance of haemophilia. A female carrier mating with a normal male will produce 50% of daughters as carriers and 50% of sons will have haemophilia (generation I). A haemophiliac male mating with a normal female will produce 100% carrier females and normal males (generation II).

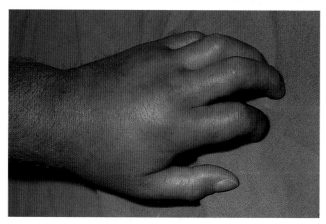

Fig. 30.2 Factor VIII deficiency: bleeding into the hand causing haematoma formation, following trauma in a patient with factor VIII deficiency.

Table 30.1 Laboratory features of inherited coagulation disorders.

Condition	PT	APTT	Bleeding time	Other
Haemophilia A	N	↑	N	Factor VIII ↓
Haemophilia B	N	↑	N	Factor IX ↓
von Willebrand's disease	N	↑	↑	von Willebrand factor ↓
				Factor VIII ↓
				Abnormal platelet aggregation with ristocetin

Complications of treatment

• HIV and hepatitis C from impure preparations (prior to the early 1980s), subsequent AIDS, hepatitis and cirrhosis.
• Neutralizing antibodies to factor VIII in 15% of severe patients may require immunosuppressive therapy, treatment with porcine factor VIII, or plasma exchange.

Factor IX deficiency (haemophilia B, Christmas disease)

Factor IX deficiency (haemophilia B, Christmas disease) has similar clinical features to haemophilia A. Also sex-linked, it is four times less common and usually milder than haemophilia A. Diagnosis and treatment are similar to haemophilia A, except that factor IX concentrate is used for treatment and desmopressin is not effective.

Von Willebrand's disease

Von Willebrand's disease is usually autosomal dominant, and results from mutations in the von Willebrand factor (vWF) gene. Von Willebrand factor is a large multimeric protein produced by endothelial cells, which carries factor VIII in plasma and mediates platelet adhesion to endothelium (see Chapter 28). The disease is more frequent than haemophilia A; males and females are affected equally.

Clinical features

• Bleeding, typically from mucous membranes (mouth, nose bleeds, menorrhagia).
• Excess blood loss following trauma or surgery.
• Haemarthroses and muscle bleeding are rare.

Diagnosis

• APTT is prolonged, PT normal.
• Factor VIII and vWF levels are reduced.
• Bleeding time is prolonged.
• Defective platelet function, reduced aggregation with ristocetin.
• Mild thrombocytopenia may occur.

Treatment

• Intermediate purity factor VIII concentrate (contains both vWF and factor VIII) for bleeding.
• Desmopressin is helpful for mild bleeding.
• Fibrinolytic inhibitors (e.g. tranexamic acid) are helpful.
• Carrier detection and antenatal diagnosis based on fetal DNA analysis is now available.

Other conditions

Factor XI deficiency has an incidence of approximately 10 cases/million population (higher among Ashkenazi Jews) and is autosomal recessive. There is poor correlation between factor XI levels and symptoms. It is generally mild, but severe spontaneous and postsurgical bleeding may occur. Congenital deficiencies of factor II, V, VII, X and XIII are rare and usually cause mild bleeding disorders. Factor XII deficiency prolongs the APTT but does not cause clinical symptoms. Fibrinogen deficiency occurs as a moderately severe autosomal recessive disorder. Dys-fibrinogenaemia (presence of a functionally abnormal molecule) is both a rare autosomal dominant disorder and a more common acquired disorder (liver disease, malignancy and systemic lupus erythematosus).

31 Disorders of coagulation II: Acquired

Liver disease

Liver disease leads to defects of coagulation, platelets and fibrinolysis.

- Reduced synthesis of vitamin K dependent factors (II, VII, IX, X, proteins C and S) caused by impaired vitamin K absorption (biliary obstruction).
- Impaired synthesis of other coagulation proteins (factor I and V).
- Thrombocytopenia (hypersplenism) and abnormal platelet function (cirrhosis).
- Fibrinolysis impaired.
- Reduced levels of proteins C and S, antithrombin and α_2 antiplasmin lead to susceptibility to disseminated intravascular coagulation (DIC).
- Dysfibrinogenaemia may lead to haemorrhage or thrombosis.

Disseminated intravascular coagulation (Fig. 31.1)

Release of procoagulant material into the circulation or endothelial cell damage causes generalized activation of the coagulation and fibrinolytic pathways leading to widespread fibrin deposition in the circulation.

Clinical features

- Both bleeding and thrombosis may occur.
- Tissue damage caused by thrombosis leads to necrosis and further activation of coagulation and fibrinolysis.
- Purpura, ecchymoses, gastrointestinal bleeding, bleeding from intravenous sites and following venepuncture may occur as a result of low levels of coagulation factors and platelets resulting from increased consumption.
- Renal function may be impaired due to microvascular thrombosis.

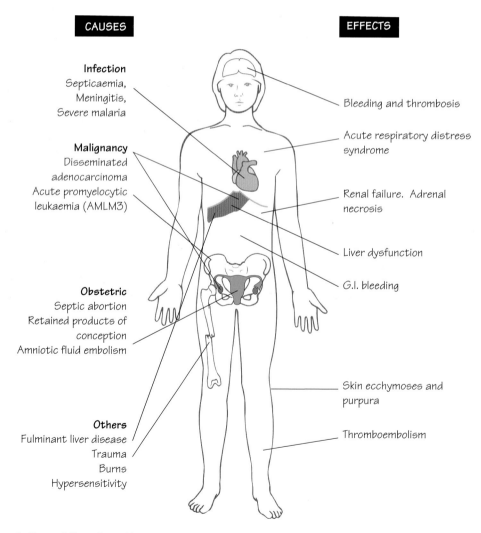

CAUSES

Infection
Septicaemia,
Meningitis,
Severe malaria

Malignancy
Disseminated
adenocarcinoma
Acute promyelocytic
leukaemia (AMLM3)

Obstetric
Septic abortion
Retained products of
conception
Amniotic fluid embolism

Others
Fulminant liver disease
Trauma
Burns
Hypersensitivity

EFFECTS

Bleeding and thrombosis

Acute respiratory distress
syndrome

Renal failure. Adrenal
necrosis

Liver dysfunction

G.I. bleeding

Skin ecchymoses and
purpura

Thromboembolism

Fig. 31.1 Causes and effects of disseminated intravascular coagulation.

Table 31.1 Coagulation changes in acquired disorders of coagulation.

	PT	APTT	TT	Platelets	Other
Liver disease	↑	↑	N/↑	↓	Dysfibrinogenaemia
DIC	↑	↑	↑	↓	FDP ↑ ±RBC fragments on blood film
Vitamin K deficiency	↑	↑ or N	N	N	
Massive transfusion	↑	↑	N	↓	
Oral anticoagulants	↑	↑	N	N	
Heparin	↑	↑	↑	N (rarely ↓)	Anti-Xa ↓

APTT, activated partial thromboplastin time; DIC, disseminated intravascular coagulation; FDP, fibrin degradation products; N, normal; PT, prothrombin time; RBC, red blood cell; TT, thrombin time.

• Other manifestations include acute respiratory distress syndrome (both a cause and complication of DIC), adrenal necrosis, shock and thromboembolism.

Laboratory features (Table 31.1)
• Thrombocytopenia.
• Nearly all tests of coagulation and fibrinolysis are abnormal with low levels of fibrinogen.
• Fibrin degradation products (e.g. X-DP or FDP) are present in plasma (X=clotting factor).
• Blood film: microangiopathic haemolytic anaemia (see Chapter 15) may occur.

Treatment
• Treat the cause, e.g. antibiotics, removal of the procoagulant stimulus (e.g. a dead fetus).
• Supportive therapy with fresh frozen plasma, platelet concentrates and cryoprecipitate if bleeding is dominant.
• Anticoagulant therapy (e.g. heparin) if thrombosis is dominant.
• Protein C and antithrombin in selected patients.

Other acquired disorders of coagulation
Drugs
• Anticoagulants and drugs affecting anticoagulation (see Chapter 33) are the most common drugs to disturb coagulation.

• Chemotherapy (e.g. L-asparaginase may lead to thrombosis).

Acquired coagulation inhibitors
These antibodies to coagulation factors are idiopathic, commoner in the elderly, or occur in malignancy (e.g. lymphoma), connective tissue disease (e.g. SLE) and with paraproteins (e.g. myeloma). They lead to excessive bleeding, both spontaneously and following injury.

Vitamin K deficiency
Vitamin K is required to activate factors II, VII, IX and X and protein C and S by γ carboxylation (see Chapter 33). It is fat-soluble and derived from vegetables in food and intestinal flora. Deficiency occurs in patients on poor diets, those taking broad-spectrum antibiotics which reduce the gut flora, in biliary tract disease and with intestinal malabsorption.

Haemorrhagic disease of the newborn
Newborn infants are at an increased risk of bleeding because of hepatic immaturity and low levels of vitamin K. It is customary to give an injection of vitamin K (1 mg) to all newborn infants in the UK. Fears that this may lead to an increased risk of cancer have not been substantiated.

32 Thrombosis and thrombophilia

Thrombosis

Thrombosis is the pathological process whereby platelets and fibrin interact with the vessel wall to form a haemostatic plug to cause vascular obstruction. It may be arterial, causing ischaemia, or venous leading to stasis (Fig. 32.1). The thrombus may be subsequently lysed by fibrinolysis, organize, recanalize or embolize. Thrombosis underlies ischaemic heart, cerebrovascular and peripheral vascular disease; venous occlusion and pulmonary embolism; and it plays an important part in pre-eclampsia.

Arterial thrombosis (Table 32.1)

This occurs in relation to damaged endothelium, e.g. atherosclerotic plaques. Exposed collagen and released tissue factor cause platelet aggregation and fibrin formation.

Venous thrombosis (Table 32.2)

Factors affecting blood flow (e.g. stasis, obesity), alterations in blood constituents and damage to vascular endothelium (e.g. caused by sepsis, surgery or indwelling catheters) are important risk factors.

Thrombophilia

Thrombophilia is a congenital or acquired predisposition to thrombosis. It should be suspected and screened for in patients who are young, have a positive family history, have a thrombosis in an unusual site and in females with recurrent fetal loss.

Inherited thrombophilia

This has been increasingly recognized recently (Tables 32.1 and 32.2; Fig. 32.2). Presentation may be during early childhood or in adulthood, e.g. at commencement of oral contraceptives or during pregnancy/puerperium. Inheritance of a variant form of factor V (factor V Leiden) is the most common (up to 5% of the population). Activated factor V Leiden is relatively resistant to inactivation by protein C. The risk of thrombosis is increased 5- to 10-fold in heterozygotes, and 50- to 100-fold in homozygotes. Rarer causes include protein C, protein S or antithrombin deficiency or functional abnormality, defective fibrinolysis (e.g. TPAI deficiency, see Chapter 28), mutant prothrombin and homocystinuria. The combination of two abnormalities often underlies severe cases.

Table 32.1 Risk factors for arterial thrombosis.

Hypertension
Smoking
Diabetes*
Hyperlipidaemia*
↑ Homocysteine*
Polycythaemia/thrombocythaemia
↑ Factor VIII
↑ Fibrinogen
Lupus anticoagulant

*May be related to an inherited abnormality.

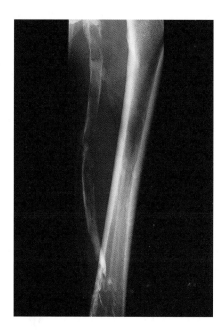

Fig. 32.1 Thrombosis: venogram showing filling defects due to a deep vein thrombus in a patient with polycythaemia.

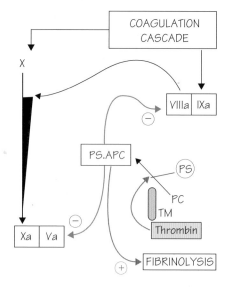

Fig. 32.2 The protein C pathway. Thrombin bound to thrombomodulin (TM) on intact endothelium activates protein C to activated protein C (APC). This combines with protein S (PS) and inactivates Va and VIIIa. Factor V Leiden is resistant to APC.

Table 32.2 Risk factors for venous thrombosis.

Conditions causing stasis

Cardiac failure, oedema, nephrotic syndrome
Postoperative
Immobility and bed rest
Trauma
Pelvic obstruction

Altered blood constituents

Coagulation factors
Hereditary
    Factor V Leiden
    Protein C deficiency
    Protein S deficiency
    Antithrombin deficiency
    Prothrombin mutation
Acquired
    Oestrogen therapy, contraceptive pill
    Malignancy
    Pregnancy and puerperium
    Lupus anticoagulant
    Raised plasma homocysteine (may also be inherited)

Blood cells
    Polycythaemia
    Thrombocythaemia

Acquired thrombophilia

Acquired hypercoagulable states are listed in Tables 32.1 and 32.2. Pathogenesis, e.g. in pregnancy, oral contraceptive pill therapy and malignancy, is multifactorial and relates to elevated levels of procoagulant factors, depressed levels of inhibitor proteins and physical factors (e.g. stasis, surgery).

Lupus anticoagulant syndrome

Despite its name, this syndrome usually presents with arterial or venous thrombosis or recurrent miscarriages. It may be associated with systemic lupus erythematosus or other connective tissue disorders, with malignancy or infections or be idiopathic. Patients may show a spectrum of antibodies which interfere with phospholipid-dependent coagulation tests *in vitro* and/or react with cardiolipin. The APTT is prolonged and not corrected by a 50:50 mix of normal plasma in patient plasma. Anticoagulant therapy is needed for patients with thrombosis.

Antiplatelet therapy

The use of heparin and warfarin is discussed in Chapter 33. Antiplatelet drugs (see Chapter 2, Fig. 2.8) and fibrinolytic drugs are discussed here.
• Aspirin (75 mg daily and 300 mg post myocardial infarc-

tion) is most widely used. It inhibits platelet function by inhibiting cyclo-oxygenase thus reducing thromboxane A_2 production.
• Others: clopidrogel and monoclonal antibodies directed to platelet glycoproteins (e.g. GP IIb/IIIa) are used, for example, post angioplasty or stent insertion.

Indications
Prevention of thrombosis in patients with:
• previous myocardial infarction, transient ischaemic attacks and stroke or high risk of first myocardial infarct in males;
• thrombocytosis, e.g. myeloproliferative disorders, post splenectomy;
• prosthetic valves and post coronary artery surgery or angioplasty;
• pre-eclampsia; and
• severe peripheral vascular disease.

Fibrinolytic therapy

This is used to enhance conversion of plasminogen to plasmin (see Chapter 28, Fig. 28.4), which degrades fibrin. It must be used within 5–7 days for venous thrombi and 5–7 h for arterial thrombi.
• Streptokinase directly activates plasminogen. Most individuals have antistreptococcal antibodies; a loading dose is therefore required and treatment becomes ineffective after 4–10 days.
• Urokinase has a similar action but may be used if there are high levels of antistreptococcal antibodies. Single chain urokinase-type plasminogen activator (SCU-PA) has also been developed.
• Acylated plasminogen streptokinase activator complex (APSAC) activates streptokinase bound to plasminogen.
• Recombinant tissue plasminogen activation (TPA) causes activation of fibrin-bound plasminogen only, and is associated with less systemic activation of fibrinolysis.

Indications
• Acute myocardial infarction: streptokinase is usually given with 300 mg aspirin and heparin intravenously.
• Treatment of arterial and venous thrombosis, e.g. pulmonary embolism, peripheral arterial or venous thrombosis.

Contraindications
• Patients with active gastrointestinal bleeding, aortic dissection, head injury or recent (<2 months) neurosurgery, and bleeding diathesis.

Side effects
• Bleeding, especially in patients taking anticoagulants or antiplatelet drugs.
• Anaphylactic reactions may occur with streptokinase.

33 Anticoagulation

Heparin

Heparin is a mucopolysaccharide which is not absorbed when given orally and is therefore given subcutaneously or intravenously. It activates antithrombin (AT) which irreversibly inactivates prothrombin, Xa, IXa and XIa. It also impairs platelet function. Unfractionated heparin (UFH) is a heterogeneous mixture of polysaccharide chains. Low-molecular-weight (LMW) heparin preparations (MW <5000) have a greater ability to inactivate Xa and less effect on thrombin (Fig. 33.1) and platelet function, and therefore have a lesser tendency to cause bleeding. They have a longer plasma half-life so that once daily subcutaneous administration is effective in prophylaxis. They also interact less than UFH with endothelium, plasma proteins, macrophages and platelets making their action more predictable.

Indications

• Acute venous thrombosis, e.g. deep vein thrombosis (DVT) and pulmonary embolism (PE). Continuous intravenous infusion of UFH for 5–7 days until warfarinized.

Subcutaneous LMW heparin is equally effective. Warfarin is usually started 1–2 days after heparin.
• Unstable angina, post myocardial infarction.
• Disseminated intravascular coagulation if this is dominated by thrombosis.
• Acute peripheral arterial occlusion.
• Prophylaxis of DVT in surgical patients, e.g. 5000 units UFH b.d. (LMW heparin 2000–5000 units once daily).
• Thrombosis prophylaxis in patients undergoing cardiac surgery or renal dialysis.
• Pregnancy. As warfarin is teratogenic, heparin is used in the first trimester of pregnancy when anticoagulation is needed.
• Maintaining patency of indwelling lines and catheters.

Monitoring

For continuous intravenous infusion, the APPT should be maintained at 1.5–2×normal. LMW heparin therapy is not normally monitored; if necessary, e.g. in renal failure or in those of very low (<50 kg) or high (>80 kg) body weight, by factor Xa assay.

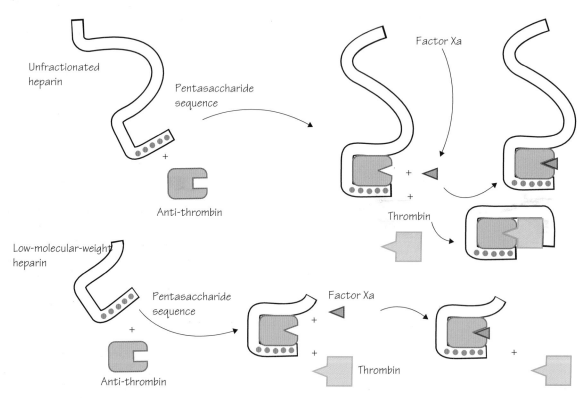

Fig. 33.1 Heparin binds to antithrombin via a pentasaccharide sequence, and induces a conformational change which allows antithrombin to bind Xa and thrombin. The shorter chain length of low molecular weight (LMW) heparin allows binding to only Xa, while unfractionated heparin will bind both Xa and thrombin. Thus, LMW heparin allows a selective inhibition of factor Xa. Modified from Weitz J.I. (1997) Low molecular-weight heparin. *New England Journal of Medicine*, **337**: 688–98.

Side effects

• Haemorrhage, particularly if combined with antiplatelet therapy, overdosage or, rarely, platelet function defect. Heparin has a short half-life (1 h); levels fall rapidly when infusion stopped. Protamine sulphate will reverse heparin immediately, but must be used with caution as it can cause haemorrhage at high dosage.
• Long-term therapy (>2 months) can lead to osteoporosis.
• Thrombocytopenia, which is antibody-mediated, may lead to platelet clumping with arterial thrombosis.
• LMW heparin is less likely to cause all these side effects.

Warfarin

Vitamin K promotes the γ carboxylation of glutamic acid residues of factor II, VII, IX and X; warfarin prevents this to cause a 50% drop of factor VII levels within 24 h and of factor II in 4 days. Full anticoagulation occurs 48–72 h after starting warfarin therapy. Non-carboxylated factors II, VII, IX and X (proteins formed in vitamin K absence, PIVKAs) appear in plasma (see Fig. 33.2). Protein C and S levels also fall and this initially (first 2–3 days) leads to an increased risk of thrombosis and may lead to skin necrosis.

Control of therapy

The PT is measured and expressed as an international normalized ratio (INR) against the mean normal PT using a calibrated thromboplastin. Treatment is monitored by maintaining the INR at 2.0–3.5, precise level depending on indication.

Indications

• Treatment of DVT, pulmonary embolism, systemic embolism (3–6 months therapy).
• Prophylaxis against thrombosis in patients with atrial fibrillation, prosthetic valves, arterial grafts, repeated pulmonary embolism and in patients with inherited or acquired predisposition and previous DVT.
• Low doses (to maintain INR 1.5) of value in prevention of myocardial infarct in high-risk groups.
• Warfarin crosses the placenta and is teratogenic in early pregnancy; heparin is given in pregnancy.

Side effects

• Haemorrhage—especially in patients taking other anti-coagulants, antiplatelet drugs or thrombolytic therapy, and in those with liver disease.

Drug interactions

Warfarin is highly bound to albumin and is metabolized by the liver. The minor unbound fraction is active. Action is increased by drugs which:

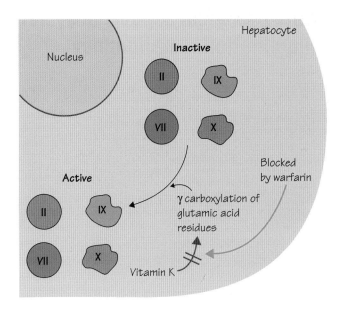

Fig. 33.2 Action of warfarin.

• reduce its binding to albumin, e.g. aspirin, sulphonamides;
• inhibit hepatic metabolism, e.g. allopurinol, tricyclic anti-depressants, sulphonamides;
• decrease absorption of vitamin K, e.g. antibiotics, laxatives;
• decrease synthesis of vitamin K factors, e.g. high-dose salicylates.
   Action is decreased by drugs which:
• accelerate its metabolism, e.g. barbiturates, rifampicin; and
• enhance synthesis of coagulation factors, e.g. oral contraceptives, hormone replacement therapy.

Reversal of action

Patients with haemorrhage and a raised INR should receive fresh frozen plasma or concentrates of factors II, VII, IX and X. If severe, also vitamin K (10 mg i.v.) but this results in resistance to warfarin for 2–3 weeks. Raised INR without haemorrhage is managed by withholding therapy for 1–2 days and repeating the INR.

Other anticoagulant drugs

The identification of thrombin receptors is likely to lead to development of receptor antagonist drugs. Hirudin (formerly purified from leech extracts, now available as a recombinant product) is a specific direct inhibitor of thrombin licensed for use in adults who cannot receive heparin (e.g. because of heparin-induced thrombocytopenia).

34 Haematological aspects of systemic disease I: Inflammation—malignancy

A wide range of abnormalities affecting red cells, white cells, platelets and coagulation factors occur in association with systemic illness.

Anaemia of chronic disease

• Anaemia of chronic disease (ACD) is a common normochromic or mildly hypochromic anaemia, occurring in patients with a systemic disease (Table 34.1). Moderate anaemia occurs (haemoglobin level >9.0 g/dL, severity of anaemia correlating with severity of underlying disease).
• Reduced serum iron and total iron binding capacity.
• Normal or raised serum ferritin with adequate iron stores in the bone marrow but stainable iron absent from erythroblasts.

Pathogenesis

Increased levels of cytokines, especially IL-1, IL-6, tumour necrosis factor and interferon-γ, which interact with accessory marrow stromal cells, macrophages and erythroid progenitors to reduce erythropoiesis, iron utilization and response to erythropoietin (EPO).

Treatment

• Therapy of the chronic disease gradually reduces levels of mediator cytokines.
• Recombinant EPO may improve anaemia in patients with, for example, rheumatoid arthritis (RA), cancer and myeloma.

Table 34.1 Conditions associated with anaemia of chronic disorders.

Chronic infections

Especially osteomyelitis, bacterial endocarditis, tuberculosis, chronic abscesses, bronchiectasis, chronic urinary tract infections, HIV, AIDS, malaria

Other chronic inflammatory disorders

Rheumatoid arthritis, polymyalgia rheumatica, systemic lupus erythematosus, scleroderma, inflammatory bowel disease, thrombophlebitis

Malignant diseases

Carcinoma, especially metastatic or associated with infection, lymphoma

Others

Congestive heart failure, ischaemic heart disease

Malignancy

Anaemia

• Anaemia of chronic disease affects almost all cancer patients at some stage.
• Blood loss in gastrointestinal and gynaecological malignancies.
• Autoimmune haemolytic anaemia (AIHA), especially in lymphoma.
• Microangiopathic haemolytic anaemia (see Chapter 15) may occur with disseminated mucin-secreting adenocarcinoma.
• Leuco-erythroblastic anaemia indicates marrow infiltration by tumour (Fig. 34.1).
• Red cell aplasia is associated with thymoma, lymphoma and chronic lymphocytic leukaemia.

Other causes

Chemotherapy or radiotherapy-induced inhibition of bone marrow. Folate deficiency as a result of poor diet and widespread disease.

Polycythaemia

Tumour cells may produce EPO or EPO-like peptides in renal cell carcinoma, hepatoma and uterine myoma (see Chapter 27).

White cell changes

Cancer patients frequently have opportunistic infections or bleed, which raises white cells (usually neutrophils), or receive chemotherapy or radiotherapy, which lowers them.

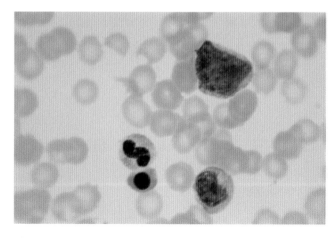

Fig. 34.1 Leuco-erythroblastic blood film showing circulating immature granulocytes and nucleated red blood cells indicating in this case marrow infiltration.

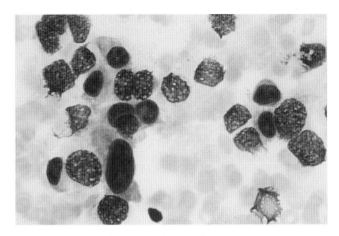

Fig. 34.2 Secondary carcinoma: bone marrow aspirate showing infiltration by breast carcinoma.

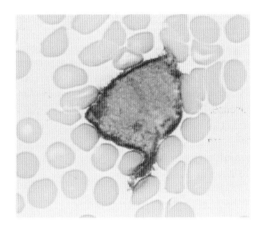

Fig. 34.3 Secondary carcinoma: bone marrow aspirate immunocytochemistry showing positive staining for cytokeratin in breast carcinoma cells.

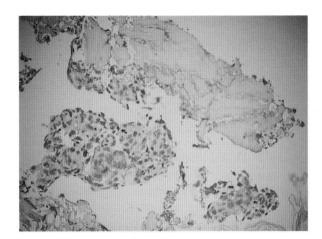

Fig. 34.4 Bone marrow trephine biopsy showing secondary carcinoma (prostatic).

Platelets
Thrombocytopenia may be due to decreased production (e.g. extensive marrow infiltration, chemotherapy or radiotherapy), accelerated peripheral destruction (e.g. disseminated intravascular coagulation, DIC) and/or hypersplenism (Figs 34.2–34.4). Immune thrombocytopenia may occur especially with lymphoma.

Thrombocytosis is a frequent reactive phenomenon in malignancy.

Coagulation changes
Activation of both coagulation and fibrinolysis may predispose to either haemorrhage or thrombosis. Chronic DIC (e.g. with pancreatic carcinoma) causes thrombosis, including migratory thrombophlebitis (Trousseau's syndrome). Circulating anticoagulants (e.g. acquired von Willebrand factor inhibitors) and specific coagulation factor inhibitors may occur.

Connective tissue disorders
Anaemia
• Anaemia of chronic disease is common. Iron deficiency may coexist in patients with gastrointestinal haemorrhage caused by non-steroidal anti-inflammatory agents.
• Autoimmune haemolytic anaemia occurs in systemic lupus erythematosus (SLE), RA and mixed connective tissue disorders (CTD).
• Red cell aplasia occurs in SLE.

White cells
Inflammation leads to neutrophilia. Neutropenia with splenomegaly occurs in patients with RA (Felty's syndrome). Antibody and immune-complex mediated neutrophil destruction and decreased neutrophil production in the marrow may also occur in SLE. Eosinophilia may occur in SLE, RA and polyarteritis nodosa.

Platelets
Thrombocytopenia may be immune (SLE, rather than scleroderma and RA). Thrombocytosis is a non-specific reactive phenomenon to inflammation in CTD.

Coagulation changes
These may be caused by associated renal disease, drug therapy, DIC and specific coagulation factor inhibitors. The lupus anticoagulant occurs in approximately 10% of patients with SLE (see Chapter 32).

35 Haematological aspects of systemic disease II: Renal, liver, endocrine—pregnancy

Renal disease
Anaemia
Acute or chronic renal failure causes a normochromic normocytic anaemia, with reduced erythropoietin (EPO) levels—the main cause of anaemia—and ecchinocytes (burr cells) in the blood film (Fig. 35.1). Iron deficiency (blood loss) and haemolysis in haemolytic uraemic syndrome and thrombotic thrombocytopenic purpura are other causes. Erythropoietin corrects anaemia up to a haemoglobin level of 12 g/dL. A poor response to EPO occurs with iron or folate deficiency, haemolysis, infection, occult malignancy, aluminium toxicity, hyperparathyroidism and inadequate dialysis. Hypertension and thrombosis of an arteriovenous fistula may occur with EPO therapy.

Polycythaemia
Polycythaemia may occur with renal tumours or cysts.

Haemostatic abnormalities
Coagulation factors II, XI or XIII may be reduced and platelet function is impaired (predispose to bleeding), whereas low levels of protein C, AT or plasminogen may lead to thrombosis.

Endocrine disease
Anaemia
Both hyper- and hypothyroidism cause mild anaemia (mean corpuscular volume, MCV, raised in hypothyroidism, low in thyrotoxicosis). Deficiencies of iron, as a result of menorrhagia or achlorhydria, or B_{12}, (increased incidence of PA in hypothyroidism, hypoadrenalism and hypoparathyroidism), may complicate the anaemia. Antithyroid drugs (carbimazole and propylthiouracil) can cause aplastic anaemia or agranulocytosis.

Liver disease
Anaemia
This may be caused by anaemia of chronic disease, haemodilution (increased plasma volume), pooling of red cells (splenomegaly) and haemorrhage (e.g. caused by oesophageal varices). The MCV is raised, particularly in alcoholics, and target cells, ecchinocytes and acanthocytes occur in the blood film (Fig. 35.2). Haemolysis and hypertriglyceridaemia with alcoholic liver disease (Zieve's syndrome) is rare. Direct toxicity of copper for red cells causes haemolysis in Wilson's disease. Viral hepatitis, including hepatitis A, B and C and hepatitis viruses yet to be characterized, may lead to aplastic anaemia. Platelets may be low (hypersplenism or DIC). Coagulation abnormalities are discussed in Chapter 31.

Platelets and haemostasis
See Table 31.1 and Chapter 31.

Haematological aspects of pregnancy
Anaemia
Plasma volume increases by up to 50% during first and second trimesters, whereas red cell mass (RCM) increases by only 20–30%. Haemodilution results (haemoglobin falls to a mean 10.5 g/dL between 16 and 40 weeks). A

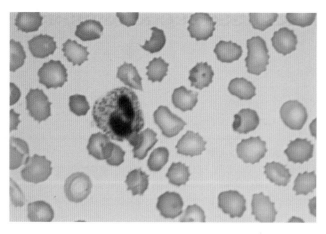

Fig. 35.1 Renal failure: peripheral blood film showing irregular red cells ('burr' cells), fragmented red blood cells and a neutrophil showing toxic granulation and vacuolation.

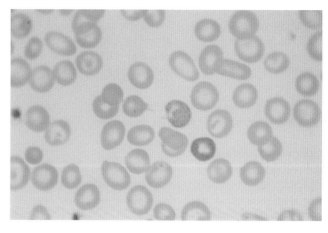

Fig. 35.2 Liver disease: peripheral blood film showing target cells, acanthocytes, macrocytes and basophilic stippling.

Table 35.1 Haemostatic changes during pregnancy.

Coagulation factors

Vitamin K dependent factors II, VII, IX, X ↑
Factor VIII ↑, von Willebrand factor ↑
Fibrinogen ↑

Coagulation inhibitors

Protein C ↑ or NC
Antithrombin ↑ or NC

Fibrinolytic activity

Reduced

DIC (see Chapter 31)

Thrombocytopenia

Gestational
Immune
Pre-eclampsia
Thrombotic thrombocytopenic purpura (typically mid trimester)
Haemolytic uraemic syndrome (typically post delivery)
Haemolytic anaemia with elevated liver enzymes and low
   platelets (HELLP) syndrome

NC, no change.

physiological rise in MCV of 5–10 fl occurs. Increase in RCM, iron transfer to the fetus and blood loss during labour together require about 1000 mg of iron, so that iron deficiency is frequent. Folate requirements rise because of increased catabolism. Early supplementation (e.g. 400 μg daily) reduces risk of megaloblastic anaemia and of fetal neural tube defects (see Chapter 12). The serum B_{12} level falls below normal in 20–30% of pregnant women, to rise again spontaneously post delivery. Autoimmune haemolytic anaemia in pregnancy is typically severe and refractory to therapy. Haemolytic anaemia with elevated liver enzymes and low platelets (HELLP syndrome) and epigastric pain may occur in the last trimester. Disseminated intravascular coagulation may accompany HELLP syndrome and induction of labour or caesarean section is often necessary.

White cells
Mild neutrophil leucocytosis with a left shift.

Platelets
Gestational thrombocytopenia complicates 8–10% of pregnancies, is mild (platelets $80–150 \times 10^9$/L) and is not associated with neonatal thrombocytopenia or significant bleeding. Maternal immune thrombocytopenic purpura may antedate pregnancy or present during it, and is associated with increased levels of platelet-associated IgG or serum platelet autoantibodies. Management includes no therapy (absence of bleeding, platelets $>50 \times 10^9$/L), corticosteroids or intravenous immunoglobulin, which also crosses placenta to elevate fetal count. Thrombocytopenia occurs in pre-eclampsia (mechanism unknown); low-dose aspirin therapy may reduce platelet consumption.

Coagulation changes
Coagulation changes (Table 35.1) combine to give an increased risk of thrombosis and DIC. This occurs in up to 40% of cases of abruptio placenta, leading to haemorrhage and shock. Retention of a dead fetus usually leads to chronic low-grade DIC with onset over 1–2 weeks. Venous stasis resulting from the gravid uterus combines with these changes to make pregnancy a hypercoagulable state; operative delivery imposes an additional risk.

36 Haematological aspects of systemic disease III: Infection, amyloid

Infections

Viruses

Anaemia

Autoimmune haemolytic anaemia may occur, especially in infectious mononucleosis, usually of cold type. B19 parvovirus causes erythema variegata or fifth disease in children and leads to transient red cell aplasia in patients with haemolytic anaemias (aplastic crisis). Anaemia occurs with pancytopenia in virus-associated bone marrow aplasia (hepatitis viruses, HIV and cytomegalovirus in organ transplant recipients). Microangiopathic haemolytic anaemia (MAHA) with thrombotic thrombocytopenic purpura (TTP) may occur.

White cells

Typically neutropenia with lymphopenia or lymphocytosis (see Chapter 8) occurs.

Platelets

Thrombocytopenia may be immune (e.g. infectious mononucleosis, HIV) caused by bone marrow aplasia, or by increased consumption—disseminated intravascular coagulation (DIC), haemophagocytosis (Fig. 36.1), haemolytic uraemic syndrome (HUS) and TTP. Reactive thrombocytosis can also occur.

Bacterial, fungal and protozoal infection

Anaemia

Anaemia of chronic disease is frequent. Haemolytic anaemia may be immune (e.g. cold antibodies with anti-I specificity in mycoplasma infection) or non-immune (e.g. direct red cell invasion, *Bartonella bacilliformis*; or toxin-mediated, *Clostridium perfringens* and *Staphylococcus aureus*). Disseminated intravascular coagulation and MAHA may occur. Haemolytic uraemic syndrome may follow infection by verotoxin-producing strains of *Escherichia coli*, *Salmonella*, *Shigella* and *Campylobacter*. Blood loss can occur with *Helicobacter pylori* and ankylostoma infections.

White cells

Neutrophilia is most common (see Chapter 8).

Platelets

Thrombocytosis is frequently reactive. Thrombocytopenia may also occur, caused by immune destruction, circulating immune complexes, decreased platelet production and DIC in severe bacterial, fungal and rickettsial infection.

Haemostasis

Disseminated intravascular coagulation may dominate the clinical picture in certain infections, e.g. bacterial meningitis.

Malaria (Fig. 36.2)

Anaemia is caused by haemolysis (cellular disruption and haemoglobin digestion), splenic sequestration, haemodilution (raised plasma volume) and ineffective erythropoiesis. Malarial antigens attached to red cells may cause immune haemolysis. Acute intravascular haemolysis with haemoglobinuria and renal failure (blackwater fever) occurs rarely in *Plasmodium falciparum* infection. Anaemia of chronic disease (ACD) may also occur. Eosinophilia is variable. Thrombocytopenia (in up to 70% of *P. falciparum* infections) may be caused by immune destruction, splenic sequestration and DIC.

Leishmaniasis

Visceral leishmaniasis is a protozoal infection caused by *Leishmania donovani*. Hepatosplenomegaly, hypergamma-

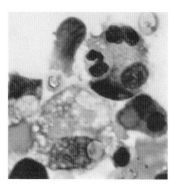

Fig. 36.1 Haemophagocytic syndrome: bone marrow aspirate showing a macrophage laden with cellular debris.

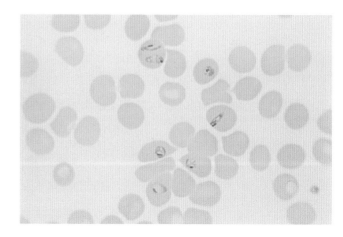

Fig. 36.2 Malaria: peripheral blood film showing red cells invaded by ring forms of *Plasmodium falciparum*.

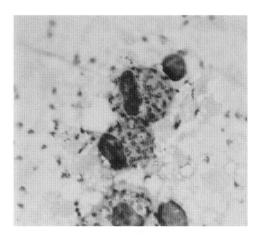

Fig. 36.3 Leishmaniasis: bone marrow aspirate showing a macrophage containing Leishman–Donovan bodies.

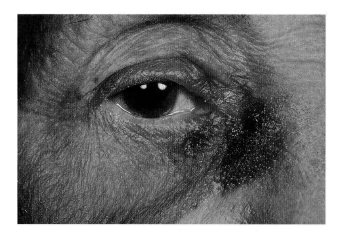

Fig. 36.4 Amyloidosis: characteristic waxy deposits around the eye.

globulinaemia, normochromic anaemia and a raised erythrocyte sedimentation rate (ESR) occur. Bone marrow aspirate shows macrophages containing Leishman–Donovan bodies (Fig. 36.3)

Amyloid

Amyloidosis is the tissue deposition of a fibrillary homogeneous eosinophilic protein material which is birefringent and stains with Congo red. It is classified into:

• amyloid derived from clonal lymphocyte or plasma cell proliferation (AL) (e.g. myeloma, primary amyloidosis) when immunoglobulin light chains or components of them are deposited (see Chapter 24); and

• reactive amyloidosis (AA) which occurs when serum amyloid A protein, an apolipoprotein, is deposited in chronic inflammatory disease (e.g. rheumatoid arthritis, inflammatory bowel disease) or chronic infection (tubercu-

losis, leprosy, osteomyelitis and bronchiectasis). Familial Mediterranean fever is a chronic inflammatory disease often affecting the kidneys and joints in which amyloidosis is a frequent complication. It is due to mutation of the pyrinin gene. The protein affects complement activation and neutrophil function.

Localized amyloid occurs in, for example, endocrine organs or skin in old age (Fig. 36.4), with deposition of protein A, hormones and other constituents.

Amyloid P protein is a serum protein related to C-reactive protein which is deposited in both AL or AA types of amyloid. Amyloid deposition leads to organ enlargement and dysfunction. Tissues involved include kidneys, heart, skin, tongue, endocrine organs, liver, spleen, gastrointestinal and respiratory tracts and the autonomic nervous system. Diagnosis is made by biopsy of tongue, gums or rectum with special staining.

37 Blood transfusion

Whole blood or plasma is collected from volunteer donors. Over 90% of the donated blood is separated to allow use of individual cell components and plasma from which specific blood products can be manufactured (Fig. 37.1).

In the UK blood donors are healthy volunteers, aged 17–70 years, who are not on medication, have had no serious previous illnesses and are at low risk for transmitting infectious agents. Drug abusers, haemophiliacs, those who have recently travelled outside Europe or lived in Africa—where malaria or AIDS may be endemic—and their sexual partners are excluded. Donors are screened for anaemia and venesected 2–3 times each year.

Donated blood is routinely tested:
• for hepatitis B and C, HIV 1 and 2, *Treponema pallidum*;
• serologically to determine the blood group (A, B or O) and Rh C, D and E type; and
• selective testing for antibodies to cytomegalovirus (CMV) is used to identify donations which are CMV-negative and thus suitable for certain patients.

Blood grouping and compatibility testing
Red cells
Red cells have surface antigens which are glycoproteins or glycolipids (Table 37.1). Individuals lacking a red cell

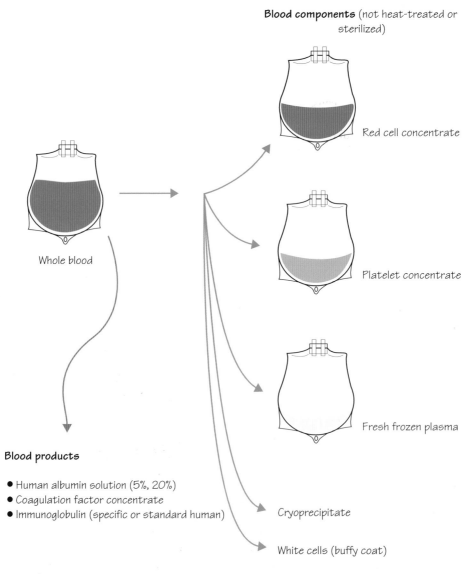

Fig. 37.1 Blood components.

Table 37.1 Red cell antigens and antibodies. Incidence in UK individuals given in brackets.

Cell antigens	Naturally occurring antibodies (usually IgM)	Antibodies only occurring after sensitization ('atypical' or immune (usually IgG))
A (40%)	Anti-B	
B (8%)	Anti-A	
AB (3%)	—	
O (45%)	Anti-A and Anti-B	
Rhesus (D) (85%)	—	
Rhesus cde/cde (i.e. Rh-negative) (15%)	—	Anti-D (Anti-C, Anti-c, Anti-E less common)
Kell (K) (9%)	—	anti-Kell
Duffy (Fya, Fyb) (60%)	—	anti-Duffy
Kidd (JKa, JKb) (75%)	—	anti-Kidd

N.B. Red cells with antigens AA or AO group as A, BB or BO group as B.

antigen may make antibodies if exposed to it by transfusion or by transfer of fetal red cells across the placenta in pregnancy. Antibodies to ABO antigens occur naturally, are IgM and complete (detectable by incubation of red cells with antibody in saline at room temperature). Antibodies to other red cell antigens appear only after sensitization. They are usually IgG and incomplete, detected by special techniques, e.g. enzyme-treated red cells, addition of albumin to the reaction mixture or the indirect antiglobulin (Coombs') reaction (see Fig. 15.2). Antibodies may cause:

• intravascular (e.g. ABO incompatibility) or extravascular (e.g. Rh incompatibility) haemolysis of donor red cells in the recipient; and
• haemolytic disease of the fetus and newborn because of transplacental passage.

Blood grouping

An individual's red cell group is determined by suspending washed red cells with diluted anti-A, anti-B, anti A+B and anti Rh (D). This is usually carried out in microtitre plates (Fig. 37.2) or gels but automated machines are increasingly used. Agglutination indicates a positive test. Serum is simultaneously incubated with group A, B and O cells to confirm the presence of the expected naturally occurring ABO antibodies. The recipient's serum is also incubated against a pool of group O cells which together express the most common antigens against which 'atypical' antibodies occur. If such an antibody is found, it is characterized. If it is clinically significant, donor blood negative for the corresponding antigen is used for transfusion.

Compatibility testing

Compatibility testing (cross-matching) entails suspension of red cells from a donor pack with recipient serum, incubation (at room temperature and 37°C) to allow reactions to occur, and examination for agglutination, including indirect antiglobulin test (see Fig. 15.2) to ensure that no reaction has occurred.

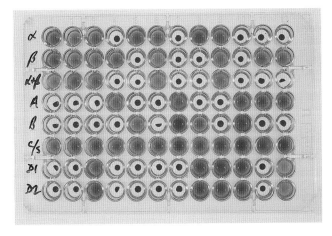

Fig. 37.2 Blood grouping of 12 subjects using microtitre plates. Agglutinated cells form a dense 'button' leaving the plasma clear. Reagents placed in the rows 1–3 are for red cell group (α = anti-A, β = anti-B, α + β = anti A + B), serum group (rows 4/5, A cells, B cells) and row 6 is a negative control (patient cells in patient serum). Rows 7 and 8 are patients' red cells with two different anti-D reagents to determine the Rh (D) group.

Red cell transfusion (Fig. 37.4a)
Indications

• Haemorrhage, severe anaemia refractory to other therapy or needing rapid correction.
• If repeated transfusions likely, phenotyped ABO and Rh (D) compatible red cells which correspond as closely as possible to the minor red cell antigens of the recipient are used to minimize sensitization.

Types of red cells

• Whole blood—for treatment of acute haemorrhage with hypovolaemia. Fresh whole blood (<5 days post collection) is preferable for neonates.
• Red cells in optimal additive solution (OAS) ('packed'), e.g. containing sodium chloride, adenine, glucose and mannitol (SAG-M) which gives red cells a shelf life of

30–35 days. These are generally used for patients with anaemia requiring red cell transfusion.

• Leucocyte-depleted red cells have been passed through a leucocyte filter either at the bedside or in the laboratory. They are given to reduce reactions to leucocytes in patients sensitized to HLA antigens (e.g. multiply transfused patients), to reduce incidence of sensitization to HLA antigens and in patients requiring CMV-negative components (e.g. CMV-negative transplant recipients, neonates/premature babies, pregnant females) when CMV status of donor is unknown. Leucodepletion reduces the theoretical risk of transmission of new variant Creutzfeldt–Jacob disease (nvCJD, see below) and all red cells in the UK are now leucodepleted.

Autologous donation

Autologous donation of red cells is suitable for some patients awaiting elective surgery. Patients donate their own red cells preoperatively on several occasions and receive iron. Donated units are screened for infectious agents in the usual way and stored at 4°C. Directed donations, e.g. within families, are not considered ethical within the UK.

Platelet transfusion (Fig. 37.4b)

A single donor unit is prepared from a unit of whole blood by centrifugation within hours of collection. It contains approximately 5×10^{10} platelets in 50–60 mL fresh plasma; shelf life of 4–6 days. Standard adult dose is five pooled units and group ABO and Rh compatible, but not cross-matched, units are given. Patients with HLA antibodies may require platelets from HLA compatible donors who have donated platelets by platelet-pheresis.

Indications

Indications for platelet transfusion are the following.
• Thrombocytopenia $<50 \times 10^9/L$—in presence of significant bleeding or prior to an invasive procedure.
• Thrombocytopenia $<10 \times 10^9/L$—prophylactic transfusions are required in patients post chemotherapy or stem cell transplant (SCT) or with failure of marrow production.
• Platelet function defects (in presence of bleeding or prior to surgery), DIC (see Chapter 31) and dilutional thrombocytopenia following massive transfusion.

White cell transfusion

White cell (buffy coat) transfusions are now rarely used in neutropenic patients as there are few data demonstrating clinical efficacy.

Fresh frozen plasma (Fig. 37.4c)

Fresh frozen plasma (FFP) is a source of all coagulation and other plasma proteins. Compatibility testing is not required, but blood group compatible units are used. Fresh frozen plasma from group AB donors may be used if the recipient blood group is unknown. As FFP is not heat sterilized and may transmit infection, solvent-treated FFP may be safer in this regard.

Indications

• Coagulation factor replacement. Perform coagulation tests and platelet count prior to use. Patients with DIC or massive transfusion at risk of bleeding and with coagulation abnormalities may benefit. Single factor deficiencies are best treated with a specific factor concentrate.
• Liver disease—in the presence of bleeding or prior to invasive procedures, e.g. liver biopsy; combined with vitamin K.
• Haemolytic uraemic syndrome or thrombotic thrombocytopenic purpura often with plasma exchange. Cryoprecipitate-poor FFP is preferred.
• Reversal of oral anticoagulation or thrombolytic therapy.

Cryoprecipitate

Cyroprecipitate is prepared from the precipitate formed from FFP during controlled thawing, resuspended in 20 mL plasma. It is rich in fibrinogen, fibronectin and factor VIII. Group compatible units are used. It may be useful in patients with DIC, liver disease, following massive transfusion and, rarely, in von Willebrand's disease.

Other blood products

These are derived from pooled human plasma which has undergone a manufacturing process designed to concentrate and sterilize the component. They carry a theoretical risk of transmitting diseases caused by prions (e.g. nvCJD). There have been no documented cases of this, but current UK practice is to use products made by recombinant DNA or plasma from non-UK donors wherever possible.

Coagulation factor concentrates

Coagulation factor concentrates are available as freeze-dried powder of high purity. Factor VIII concentrate is used for treatment of haemophilia A and von Willebrand's disease; recombinant factor VIII is now available. Factor IX concentrate, also available as recombinant, is used in patients with haemophilia B. Factor IX complex (prothrombin complex) also contains factors II, VII and X and is of value in patients with specific disorders involving factors II and X, oral anticoagulant overdose, in severe liver failure and to overcome inhibitors to factor VIII in patients with haemophilia A who have developed inhibitors. Its use carries a risk of provoking thrombosis and DIC.

Other concentrates include protein C, antithrombin, factors VII, XI and XIII and are used in the corresponding congenital deficiencies.

Albumin solution

Albumin solution is available as 5%, 20% and 20% salt-poor formulations. It contains no coagulation factors. It is used in the treatment of hypovolaemia, particularly when caused by burns, and shock associated with multiple organ failure. Synthetic plasma volume expanders (e.g. dextrans, gelatin and hydroxyethyl starch) are of equal value in initial management. These 'colloids' remain longer within the intravascular space than 'crystalloid' solutions (e.g. 0.9% NaCl), exert a colloid osmotic effect and may elevate blood pressure. Resistant oedema in patients with renal and hepatic disease requires 20% albumin.

Immunoglobulins

Immunoglobulins (Igs) are prepared from pooled donor plasma by fractionation and sterile filtration. Specific Igs include hepatitis B and herpes zoster which provide passive immune protection. Standard human Ig for intramuscular injection is used for prophylaxis against hepatitis A, rubella and measles, whereas hyperimmune globulin is prepared from donors with high titres of the relevant antibodies for prophylaxis of tetanus, hepatitis A, diphtheria, rabies, mumps, measles, rubella, CMV and *Pseudomonas* infections. Intravenous Ig may be used to protect against infections in patients with congenital or acquired immune deficiency and is of value in some autoimmune disorders, e.g. immune thrombocytopenic purpura.

Complications of transfusion (see Table 37.2)

• **Administrative and clerical errors** must be avoided by rigorous adherence to procedures for checking and documentation when ordering, prescribing, issuing and administering blood components. **These are by far the most common cause of serious and 'near miss' incidents.**
• **Congestive heart failure** caused by circulatory overload.
• **Immunological reactions** may occur with transfusion of cellular and plasma derived blood components. ABO incompatible red cell transfusions may lead to life-threatening intravascular haemolysis of transfused cells with fever, rigors, haemoglobinuria, hypotension and renal failure. Atypical antibodies arising from previous transfusions or pregnancy may cause intravascular or, more commonly, delayed extravascular haemolysis with anaemia, jaundice, splenomegaly and fever.

Hypersensitivity reactions to plasma components may cause urticaria, wheezing, facial oedema and pyrexia but can cause anaphylactic shock, especially in IgA-deficient subjects.

Treatment

The transfusion must be stopped immediately. For severe reactions, the clerical details must be checked and samples from the donor unit and recipient are analysed for compatibility and haemolysis. Recipient serum is analysed for presence of atypical red cell, leucocyte, HLA and plasma protein antibodies. Support care to maintain blood pressure and renal function, to promote diuresis and treat shock (intravenous steroids, antihistamines, adrenaline in severe cases) may be necessary.
• **Transmission of infection.** *Bacterial infections* can occur through failure of sterile technique at time of collection or because of bacteraemia in the donor. *Protozoal infections* (e.g. malaria) can be transmitted and at-risk donors are not

Table 37.2 Complications of blood transfusion.

---

1 Administrative and clerical errors leading to incompatibility between donor and recipient

2 Circulatory overload

Congestive heart failure

3 Immunological reactions

Haemolytic transfusion reactions
    Immediate, e.g. ABO compatibility
    Delayed, e.g. Rh incompatibility
Non-haemolytic transfusion reactions
    Caused by HLA antibodies
    Caused by hypersensitivity to plasma components

4 Transmission of microbial disease

Bacterial, e.g. *Yersinia*
Protozoal, e.g. malaria
Viral
    Plasma-borne viruses
    Hepatitis B + variants
    Hepatitis A (rarely)
    Other unidentified hepatitis viruses
    HIV-1 and HIV-2 (also cellular)
    Parvovirus
Cell associated viruses
    Cytomegalovirus
    Epstein–Barr virus
    HTLV-I and HTLV-II

5 Iron overload

6 Other complications

Immune deficiency, graft vs. host disease

7 Complications of massive transfusion

Hypothermia, disseminated intravascular coagulation, thrombocytopenia, electrolyte disturbance
Transfusion-associated lung injury

Hepatitis B vaccine should be given to HBV-negative recipients of pooled plasma products or patients requiring repeated red cell transfusion.

eligible to donate. *Viral infection* can be transmitted in spite of mandatory screening, as seroconversion may not have occurred in an infected donor, the virus may not have been identified, or the most sensitive serological tests may not be routinely performed (e.g. testing for antihepatitis B core antibodies). The risk of transmission is much lower for those blood products which have undergone a manufacturing and sterilization process. There is a theoretical risk of transmitting prion diseases, e.g. nvCJD, by plasma products (see above).

• **Other complications.** Iron overload occurs in multiply transfused patients (see Chapter 10). Graft vs. host disease may be caused by transfusion of viable T lymphocytes into severely immunosuppressed hosts so cellular components should be irradiated prior to transfusion to fetuses, premature neonates, SCT recipients and other severely immunocompromised patients.

Haemolytic disease of the fetus and newborn

Haemolytic disease of the fetus and newborn (HDFN) is the haemolysis of fetal or neonatal red cells caused by transplacental passage of maternal red cell antibodies (Fig. 37.3).

HDFN caused by ABO antibodies

Although ABO incompatibility between mother and fetus is common, this type of HDFN is rarely severe. Most ABO antibodies are IgM and therefore cannot cross the placenta. Fetal A and B antigens are not fully developed at birth and the maternal antibodies can be partially neutralized by A

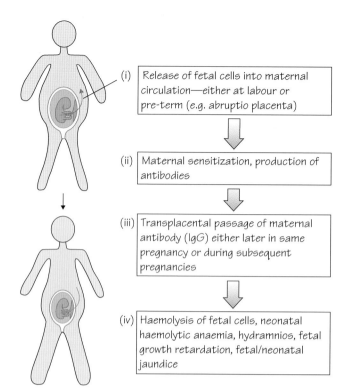

(i) Release of fetal cells into maternal circulation—either at labour or pre-term (e.g. abruptio placenta)

(ii) Maternal sensitization, production of antibodies

(iii) Transplacental passage of maternal antibody (IgG) either later in same pregnancy or during subsequent pregnancies

(iv) Haemolysis of fetal cells, neonatal haemolytic anaemia, hydramnios, fetal growth retardation, fetal/neonatal jaundice

Fig. 37.3 Haemolytic disease of the fetus and newborn (HDFN).

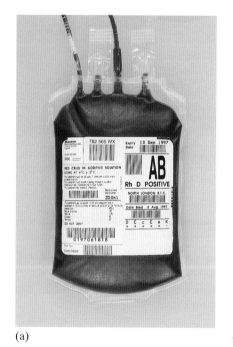

(a)

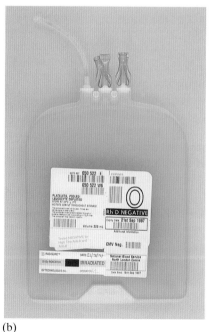

(b)

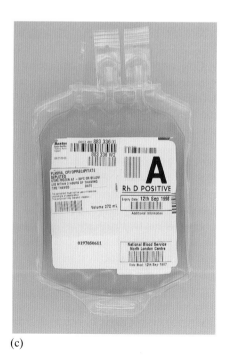

(c)

Fig. 37.4 (a) Red cells, (b) platelet pool, (c) fresh frozen plasma.

and B antigens present on other cells, in the plasma and in tissue fluids.

HDFN caused by other antibodies

The most important cause is anti-D, produced in Rh (D)-negative women as a result of sensitization during a previous pregnancy or blood transfusion and causing haemolysis in Rh (D)-positive infants. Other important causes are other antibodies within the Rh system (e.g. anti-c), anti-Kell, anti-Duffy and anti-JKa antibodies.

Haemolysis of fetal cells can lead to hydrops fetalis, though nowadays it more commonly leads to neonatal haemolytic anaemia. All women must have their blood group determined at booking and atypical red cell antibodies in plasma should be detected. If present, their titre is monitored throughout pregnancy. Ultrasound for fetal growth, fetal blood sampling and measurements of bilirubin levels in amniotic fluid are used to monitor fetal well-being.

Treatment

Transfusion of CMV-negative irradiated red cells compatible with maternal serum may be given to fetuses. Maternal antibody levels can be lowered by plasma exchange. Phototherapy and exchange transfusion of the neonate allows removal of unconjugated bilirubin which may otherwise deposit in the basal ganglia to cause neurological sequelae (kernicterus).

Prevention

Prevention is by administration of anti-D to unsensitized Rh (D)-negative women within 72 h of a potentially sensitizing event (e.g. birth of an Rh (D)-positive fetus, abortion or antepartum haemorrhage). The anti-D will coat fetal cells which are then removed from the maternal circulation before sensitization occurs. The dosage of anti-D is adjusted according to the number of fetal cells detected in the maternal circulation (Kleihauer test). All Rh (D)-negative women are now given anti-D at 28 and 34 weeks routinely.

38 Stem cell transplantation

Stem cell transplantation (SCT) (Fig. 38.1) is the use of haemopoietic stem cells (HSC) from a donor harvested from peripheral blood (peripheral blood stem cells, PBSC) or bone marrow, to repopulate recipient bone marrow.

- **Allogeneic** SCT involves transplantation of HSC from one individual to another. This is usually between two HLA matching individuals, most frequently siblings but, in their absence, volunteer and HLA matched unrelated donors (MUD) are increasingly being used. HLA matching includes class I (A,B tested serologically) and class II (DR tested serologically or by molecular typing). If the donor is an identical twin, the transplant is termed 'syngeneic'. 'Mini' transplants in which the recipient receives immunosuppressive but not myeloablative therapy are currently being explored. Pre-transplant conditioning is less intensive and the procedure is likely to be safer in older patients.
- **Autologous** SCT utilizes the patient's own stem cells. These are harvested from the patient then used to repopulate the marrow after further high-dose chemotherapy and/or radiotherapy.
- **Cord** blood transplantation utilizes fetal stem cells harvested at the time of birth from the umbilical cord.

Allogeneic SCT is rarely performed in individuals >55 years of age, as it carries risk of treatment-related morbidity and even mortality (up to 5–10%) which increases with age. Autologous SCT may be performed more safely in older patients, up to 70 years.

Indications (Table 38.1)

Stem cell transplantation is used to 'rescue' the patient from bone marrow failure or following intensive chemotherapy (± radiotherapy). For allogeneic SCT the recipient requires 'conditioning' therapy (chemotherapy ± radiotherapy) pre-transplant to cause immunosuppression, thereby reducing risk of marrow rejection, and to eradicate malignant disease in bone marrow and elsewhere. The transplanted immune system in an allogeneic SCT may itself have antitumour, e.g. graft vs. leukaemia (GVL) effect.

Procedure

Treatment with a haemopoietic growth factor (e.g. G-CSF), combined in the case of autologous SCT with chemotherapy, e.g. high-dose cyclophosphamide, is used to mobilize HSC from bone marrow into peripheral blood, where they are collected by leucopheresis. Alternatively, HSC may be harvested from marrow by multiple bone marrow aspirations, performed under general anaesthesia. Approximately 2×10^8/kg nucleated cells or 2×10^6/kg CD34 cells are needed (CD34 is a surface marker of early haemopoietic stem and progenitor cells). The recipient of an allogeneic or MUD transplant then receives immunosuppressive drugs to reduce the risk of graft vs. host disease (GVHD) (see below).

Complications

Complications of SCT include the following.
- Side effects of conditioning chemotherapy/radiotherapy, e.g. bone marrow failure, nausea, alopecia, skin burns, pulmonary toxicity, hepatic veno-occlusive disease, toxicity to endocrine organs and growth retardation.
- Rejection of transplanted HSC.
- Relapse of original disease. This is sometimes treated by infusion of lymphocytes from the allogeneic donor, which will have a GVL effect.
- Infection following SCT occurs because patients are severely immunosuppressed. Infection may be bacterial, viral, protozoal or fungal. Prophylactic antibiotics, antifungal and antiviral therapy is given. CMV-negative recipients should receive blood components which are leucodepleted or from CMV-negative donors. CMV infection may cause pneumonitis, diarrhoea, liver dysfunction, skin rash and graft failure, and is a major cause of transplant-related mortality. Ganciclovir and foscarnet are useful in treatment of CMV infection. Prophylaxis against *Pneumocystis carinii* infection is with oral co-trimoxazole and/or nebulized pentamidine.

Table 38.1 Indications for stem cell transplantation.

Allogeneic	Autologous
Acute leukaemia	**Selected patients**
Standard/poor risk AML in	
first remission	Multiple myeloma
AML in second remission	Lymphoma
Poor risk childhood or adult ALL in	Acute leukaemia
first remission	Autoimmune disease
ALL in second remission	e.g. scleroderma
Chronic or accelerated phase CML	
Severe aplastic anaemia	

Selected patients

Myelodysplasia
Lymphoma
Myeloma
Chronic lymphocytic leukaemia
Thalassaemia major, sickle cell disease
Severe inherited metabolic diseases, e.g. adenosine deaminase
  deficiency, Hurler's syndrome

ALL, acute lymphoblastic leukaemia; AML, acute myeloid leukaemia; CML, chronic myeloid leukaemia.

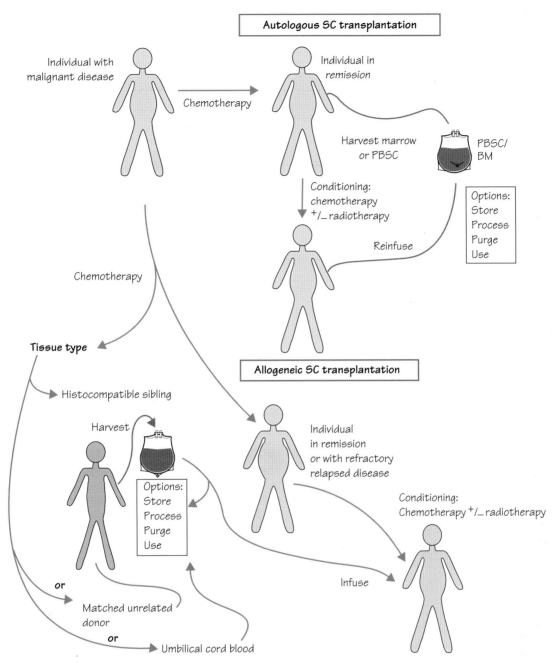

Fig. 38.1 Stem cell transplantation. Harvested stem cells may be frozen and stored indefinitely. They may be 'processed', for example to concentrate CD34 cells or remove T cells. Procedures are available to 'purge' them of residual malignant cells (e.g. by use of monoclonal antibodies).

• Metabolic problems, often caused by multiple intravenous drugs (antibiotics, antivirals, antifungals), renal failure, blood component therapy, intravenous feeding, etc.
• Graft vs. host disease (GVHD) (allogeneic SCT). Transplanted lymphocytes may recognize the recipient as 'foreign' and mount an immunological onslaught, to cause skin rash, liver disease and diarrhoea. The incidence of GVHD is higher in older patients. Acute GVHD (<100 days after SCT) typically begins 7–10 days after transplantation and is graded according to severity. Chronic GVHD (>100 days) presents with a scleroderma-like syndrome, liver, lung, gastrointestinal or joint abnormalities. The incidence and severity of GVHD may be decreased by depleting T cells from donor marrow and immune suppression of the recipient.

39 General aspects of treatment

Chemotherapy

Chemotherapy is the use of pharmacological agents (Table 39.1) to treat malignant or other proliferative diseases. It may be given orally, by bolus, prolonged subcutaneous or intravenous injection/infusion or intrathecally. It may be a single agent or combination chemotherapy utilizing drugs with different, preferably synergistic, modes of action, with limited or no overlapping toxicity, and aimed at delaying emergence of drug resistance. Chemotherapy drugs are often given as a cycle of a few days' treatment every 3–6 weeks to allow normal cells, especially of the bone marrow and gastrointestinal tract, to recover from toxicity. Extravasation into tissues can cause severe local reactions. Intravenous chemotherapy is usually given through a central line or through a tunnelled intravenous catheter (e.g. Hickman's) or indwelling chamber (e.g. Porta-Cath).

Side effects of chemotherapy

Most chemotherapeutic agents are toxic to normal dividing cells (gastrointestinal tract, haemopoietic cells, hair, skin) as well as to malignant cells. Common side effects include the following.
• Bone marrow failure (anaemia, thrombocytopenia, leucopenia) with increased susceptibility to bleeding and infection, which may require therapy with antimicrobials, blood components and recombinant growth factors (G-CSF, GM-CSF, thrombopoietin, erythropoietin).

Table 39.1 Chemotherapy agents.

DNA binding	Antimetabolites
Anthracyclines	Methotrexate
Daunorubicin	Mercaptopurine
Hydroxydaunorubicin	Thioguanine
Idarubicin	Cytosine arabinoside
Other	Hydroxyurea
Mitoxantrone	
Bleomycin	**Inhibitors of DNA repair enzymes**
	Epipodophyllotoxins
Alkylating agents	
	Antipurines
Cyclophosphamide	
Ifosphamide	Fludarabine
Chlorambucil	Deoxycoformycin
Melphalan	2-Chlorodeoxyodenosine
Nitrosoureas (BCNU, CCNU)	
Busulphan	**Others**
	Corticosteroids
Mitotic inhibitors	L-Asparaginase
	Biological agents
Vincristine	
Vindesine	
Vinblastine	

• Nausea and vomiting, requiring antiemetic therapy—metoclopramide, dexamethazone and 5-HT antagonists (e.g. ondansetron, granisetron).
• Mucositis (sore mouth and throat), abdominal pain and diarrhoea.
• Infertility—sperm storage considered *before* chemotherapy.
• Tumour lysis syndrome—prevented by good hydration, alkalinization of urine, allopurinol.
• Hyperuricaemia—prevented by allopurinol.
• Specific side effects of chemotherapy include: neuropathy (vincristine), cardiomyopathy (anthracyclines), thrombosis (L-asparaginase), secondary leukaemia (alkylating agents, etoposide), pulmonary fibrosis (busulphan) and haemorrhagic cystitis (cyclophosphamide).

Mechanism of action

Chemotherapy drugs generally affect DNA synthesis or repair and promote cellular apoptosis. Cycle-specific agents prevent DNA synthesis and act on the S phase of the cell cycle (Table 39.1). Non-cycle-specific agents act at all phases of the cell cycle and include alkylating agents, which bind to DNA, and anthracyclines, which cause DNA strand breaks. Inhibition of the DNA repair enzyme, topoisomerase II, is an important component of the action of anthracyclines and etoposide.

Biological therapies

Growth factors in clinical use (see Chapter 1) include G-CSF and GM-CSF (Fig. 39.1), and erythropoietin. The interferons are naturally occurring agents which have both antineoplastic and anti-infective properties. Interferon-α is used in treatment of chronic myeloid leukaemia, multiple myeloma, and non-Hodgkin lymphoma. Monoclonal antibodies alone or bound to toxins or radioactive isotopes may be used to kill specific cells or target drug therapy.

Infection

The main risk factors are:
• neutropenia (particularly if $<0.5\times10^9$/L) for bacterial and fungal infections;
• defective cell-mediated or humoral immunity for viral, bacterial and atypical infections (e.g. tuberculosis);
• others, such as indwelling catheters (intravenous, urethral), corticosteroid therapy and mucositis also increase risk. Impaired splenic function or splenectomy reduce ability to make antibody, particularly to capsulated organisms, reduces clearance of intracellular organisms (e.g. parasitized red cells) and impairs defence against organisms and toxins in the portal circulation. Organisms which

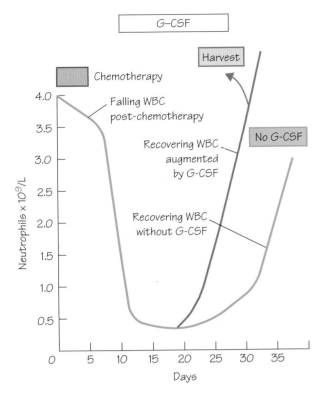

Fig. 39.1 The use of the growth factor G-CSF accelerates recovery of the white cell count after chemotherapy. It also affects granulocyte function; GM-CSF may have a particular role in treatment of fungal infections.

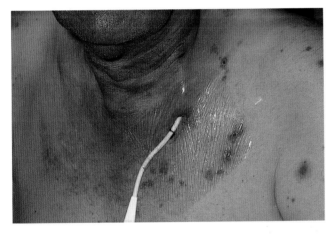

Fig. 39.2 Acute leukaemia: Hickman line infection, which has rapidly evolved to septicaemia, and bloodborne skin lesions caused by coagulase-negative staphylococci.

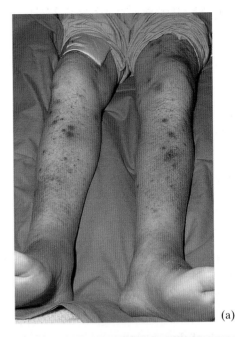

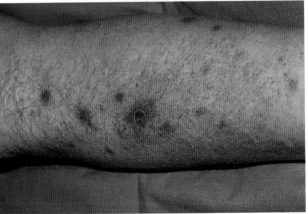

Fig. 39.3 Septicaemia in acute leukaemia leading to infected skin lesions.

are normal commensals may be pathogenic for immuno-compromised patients.

Organisms

Organisms include the following:

• bacterial—Gram-positive (coagulase-negative and -positive staphylococci, streptococci, enterococci); Gram-negative (klebsiella, pseudomonas, *Escherichia coli*, proteus); others, e.g. tuberculosis, atypical mycobacteria (Figs 39.2 and 39.3);
• fungal—*Candida*, aspergillus;
• viruses—cytomegalovirus, herpesviruses, adenoviruses; and
• protozoans—toxoplasma, pneumocystis, Leishmania, histoplasma.

Prevention

• Good hygiene on the part of the patient and staff, regular hand cleaning and avoidance of contact with infected individuals.

- Barrier nursing in isolation is preferred. Staff wear gowns and gloves when in contact with severely neutropenic patients.
- Filtered air at positive pressure reduces risk from fungal spores.
- Food should ideally be cooked. Foods frequently contaminated with bacteria (soft cheeses, uncooked eggs and meat, salads, live yoghurt) are avoided and only peeled fruits are allowed.
- Oral non-absorbable antibiotics (e.g. neomycin, colistin) will reduce colonization of the gastrointestinal tract, oral systemic antibiotics (ciprofloxacin, co-trimoxazole) reduce the incidence of bacteraemia and oral anti-fungals (fluconazole/amphotericin/itraconozole) and/or oral antiviral (acyclovir) prophylaxis are routinely given in some units.

Diagnosis

- Fever is the cardinal sign of infection: tachycardia, tachypnoea, fall in blood pressure, cough, dysuria, altered mental state may also occur.
- Physical signs include reddened throat, inflamed intravenous catheter site, skin rash, chest signs, mouth signs and perineal inflammation. Pus is absent in neutropenic patients.
- Special tests to identify the responsible organism include microbial culture (sputum, urine, throat and perineal swab, blood cultures from peripheral blood and indwelling catheter, lumbar puncture—if neurological symptoms—skin swabs, faecal culture). Bronchoalveolar lavage may be necessary. Serological tests for specific organisms, e.g. aspergillus, may be of value. Imaging tests may include chest X-ray, CT scan, especially of chest if fungal infection is suspected, and sinus X-rays.

Treatment

- Supportive care for renal failure/hypotension/respiratory failure.
- Empirical antibacterial therapy should be commenced in patients who are neutropenic ($<0.5\times10^9$/L) or otherwise severely immunocompromised and develop fever (temperature of 38°C or greater lasting for more than 2 hours). Cultures should be taken and intravenous antibiotics should be commenced, with either a single, potent broad-spectrum agent (e.g. a fourth generation cephalosporin or ureidopenicillin) or a combination of agents with activity against gram negative and gram positive (including coagulase negative staphylococci) organisms.

Radiotherapy

Ionizing radiation, usually derived from an external source, is used to treat disease by causing DNA damage in malignant cells. It is commonly used in the treatment of haematological malignancies (e.g. lymphoid leukaemias, lymphoma, myeloma) and as part of conditioning therapy for bone marrow transplant for malignant disease. Side effects include nausea, vomiting, alopecia, bone marrow failure, damage to normal tissues (e.g. skin burns), growth retardation and induction of second malignancies.

Other therapies

Blood and blood component therapy are discussed in Chapter 37. Splenectomy is beneficial in a number of haematological conditions, particularly when the spleen is the site of excessive destruction of peripheral blood cells (e.g. selected patients with haemolytic anaemia and thrombocytopenia (particularly auto-immune), myelofibrosis). The spleen has an important role in removing opsonized bacteria (see Chapter 3) and splenectomy (or hyposplenism due to disease, e.g. sickle cell disease) can lead to an increased susceptibility to infection. The operation should be avoided in children under 5 years and should be preceded by vaccination against pneumococcus, haemophilus influenza type B and meningococcus. Patients who are hyposplenic or post-splenectomy should take prophylactic antibiotics indefinitely (e.g. oral Penicillin V or erythromycin at low dose) and should at all times carry a card informing them and their carers of their condition.

Counselling

Counselling is valuable for various groups of haematological patients.

- Patients and families with malignant disease need emotional support during treatment and/or bereavement. Practical help with housing, transport, welfare benefits, etc. There should be good liaison with GPs, terminal care support teams in the community and hospices.
- Genetic counselling is needed in families with haemophilia, thalassaemia, sickle cell disease and related conditions.

Appendix I: Cluster of differentiation nomenclature system

Cell surface markers are molecules in the cell membrane that can be recognized by reactivity with specific monoclonal antibodies. Their presence gives information about the lineage, function or stage of development of a particular cell population. The cluster of differentiation (CD) nomenclature system groups together antibodies recognizing the same surface molecule (antigen).

Table A1 T-cell markers.

CD no.	Remarks
1 a, b, c	Thymocytes, Langerhans' cells (CD1a)
2	E-rosette receptor. All T cells
3	T-cell receptor. Mature T cells
4	T helper/inducer subset
5	T cells (aberrantly expressed in B-CLL, mantle cell lymphoma)
7	T cells (aberrantly expressed in some AML)
8	T cytotoxic/suppressor

Table A2 B-cell markers.

CD no.	Remarks
19	B cells, including early B cells
20	Mature B cells
21	Mature B cells. C3d receptor, EBV receptor
22	B cells
23	Activated B cells

Table A3 Myeloid and other markers.

CD no.	Remarks
Myeloid markers	
11a, 11b, 11c	Adhesion molecule ligand. Also expressed on some B and T cells and monocytes
13	All mature myeloid cells
33	Myelin-associated protein. Early myeloid cells
Others	
14	Monocytes, macrophages
25	IL2 receptor-activated B cells
34	Stem cells
45	Leucocyte common antigen: all haemopoietic cells
56	Natural killer cells
9, 29, 31, 41, 42	Platelet markers
38	Plasma cell marker
71	Red cell precursors
TdT	Terminal deoxynucleotidyl transferase — early B- and T-cell precursors

Appendix II: Further reading

Bain B.J. (1995) *Blood Cells: A Practical Guide* (2nd edn). Blackwell Science, Oxford.

Hoffbrand A.V. & Pettit J.E. (2000) *Clinical Atlas of Haematology* (3rd edn). Mosby, London.

Hoffbrand A.V., Pettit J.E. & Moss P.A. (2000) *Essential Haematology* (4th edn). Blackwell Science, Oxford.

Hoffbrand A.V., Lewis S.M. & Tuddenham E.G.D. (eds) (1999) *Postgraduate Haematology* (4th edn). Butterworth-Heinemann, Oxford.

Hoffman R., Benz E.J., Shattil S.J., Furie B., Cohen M.J. & Silberstein L.E. (1995) *Hematology: Basic Principles and Practice* (2nd edn). Churchill Livingstone, New York.

Lee G.R., Foerster J., Lukens J.N., Paraskevas F. & Rodgers G. (eds) (1998) *Wintrobe's Clinical Hematology* (10th edn). Lippincott, Williams & Wilkins, Philadelphia.

Mehta A.B. (1995) *Self Assessment Colour Review of Haematology*. Manson Publishing, London.

Appendix III: Sample questions and case histories

Questions

1 Iron deficiency anaemia.
   (a) Is usually associated with a raised MCV.
   (b) The MCH is usually low.
   (c) Is most commonly due to dietary deficiency.
   (d) Is associated with a low serum ferritin.
   (e) Responds much more quickly to parenteral than oral therapy.

2 Macrocytic anaemia
   (a) Occurs in renal failure.
   (b) May result from vitamin B12 deficiency.
   (c) Occurs in the context of chronic inflammatory disease.
   (d) May be associated with myxoedema.
   (e) May be associated with thalassemia.

3 Chronic myeloid leukaemia
   (a) Is the commonest form of leukaemia worldwide.
   (b) Usually presents with bone marrow failure.
   (c) Is usually associated with the presence of the Philadelphia chromosome.
   (d) May respond to treatment with interferon.
   (e) Usually transforms to an acute leukaemia.

4 Chronic lymphocytic leukaemia
   (a) Is a cause of hypogammaglobulinaemia.
   (b) Is commonly treated with intensive combination chemotherapy.
   (c) Is associated with a median survival of <2 years.
   (d) Often presents asymptomatically.
   (e) Is more commonly derived from B cells than T cells.

5 The myelodysplastic syndrome (MDS)
   (a) May occur as a result of prior chemotherapy.
   (b) Is thought to have a viral aetiology.
   (c) May be associated with the presence of sideroblastic anaemia.
   (d) May be associated with pancytopenia.
   (e) Is characterized by a reduction in the circulating monocyte count.

6 With regard to anticoagulant therapy
   (a) Warfarin is safer than heparin in pregnancy.
   (b) The INR is used to control heparin therapy.
   (c) Low molecular weight heparin can be given orally.
   (d) Vitamin K is used to reverse the action of warfarin.
   (e) Should be undertaken lifelong after a single pulmonary embolus.

7 Fresh frozen plasma
   (a) Is recommended in the treatment of haemophilia A.
   (b) Is heat treated and therefore free from risk of transmission of viral disease.
   (c) Is useful in the treatment of immune thrombocytopenia.
   (d) Is useful in the treatment of thrombotic thrombocytopenic pupura.
   (e) Must be prepared from whole blood within a few hours of donation.

8 Neonatal thrombocytopenia
   (a) Can occur in infants of mothers with immune thrombocytopenia.
   (b) Is often due to intrauterine viral infection.
   (c) May be due to transplacental passage of anti-platelet antibodies from the mother.
   (d) Often improves spontaneously.
   (e) May be associated with absent radii.

9 Haemolytic anaemia
   (a) Occurs whenever red cell survival is reduced.
   (b) Is often accompanied by an increase in serum unconjugated bilirubin.
   (c) Is usually accompanied by increased urinary bilirubin.
   (d) Is predominantly extravascular in hereditary spherocytosis.
   (e) Can lead to kernicterus in the neonate.

10 An increase in peripheral blood eosinophils (eosinophilia)
   (a) Is commonly seen in bacterial infection.
   (b) May be an indicator of drug hypersensitivity.
   (c) Is commonly seen in myeloproliferative disorders.
   (d) Can lead to cardiomyopathy.
   (e) Can occur in connective tissue disorders.

11 Haematological changes during normal pregancy include
   (a) An increase in MCV.
   (b) An increased incidence of thalassaemia trait.
   (c) Increased circulating levels of factor VIII.
   (d) Neutrophilia.
   (e) Increased platelet count.

12 Polycythaemia rubra vera
   (a) Occurs more frequently in smokers.
   (b) May present as gout.
   (c) Many transform to acute leukaemia.
   (d) Is frequently associated with raised white cell and platelet counts.
   (e) Is associated with an enlarged spleen.

13 Platelets
   (a) Are an important source of thrombin.
   (b) Are often multinucleated.
   (c) Are often increased in number in pateints with iron deficiency.
   (d) Will aggregate in response to ADP.
   (e) Are sometimes reduced in number in von Willebrand's disease.

14 Haemopoietic stem cells
   (a) Are derived from the thymus.
   (b) Circulate in peripheral blood.
   (c) Are progenitors for plasma cells.

(d) Do not express the CD34 antigen.
(e) Decline in number with increasing age.

15 With regard to autosomal recessive conditions
 (a) Glucose-6-phosphate dehydrogenase deficiency is an example.
 (b) Hereditary spherocytosis is an example.
 (c) There is a 1:2 chance that the offspring of two carriers will be homozygous.
 (d) The carrier state may be associated with a small survival advantage.
 (e) There is usually a disease related mutation within a single gene.

16 The following are known to cause aplastic anaemia
 (a) Chloramphenicol therapy.
 (b) Malaria.
 (c) Amyloidosis.
 (d) Viral hepatitis.
 (e) Renal cysts.

17 With regard to stem cell transplantation (SCT)
 (a) Allogeneic SCT is indicated for all patients with AML in first remission who have an HLA-identical sbiling.
 (b) Matched unrelated donor (MUD) transplantation is contra-indicated in children.
 (c) The incidence of graft versus host disease (GVHD) is reduced by depletion of T cells from the graft.
 (d) Donor stem cells are irradiated to reduce GVHD.
 (e) EBV infection is a major cause of post transplant mortality.

18 The non-Hodgkin lymphomas
 (a) Are more likely to be T cell than B cell lineage.
 (b) Occur more frequently in patients with HIV infection.
 (c) Are more likely to be disseminated (stage IV) when the histology is of indolent disease than when histology shows aggressive disease.
 (d) Are commoner than Hodgkin lymphoma.
 (e) Are declining in incidence.

19 The following are risk factors for thrombosis
 (a) Haemophilia B.
 (b) Resistance is activated protein C.
 (c) Nephrotic syndrome.
 (d) Raised levels of plasma homocysteine.
 (e) Paroxysmal nocturnal haemoglobinuria.

20 Important causes of humoral immunodeficency include
 (a) Pyruvate kinase deficiency.
 (b) Multiple myeloma.
 (c) Indolent non-Hodgkin lymphoma.
 (d) Lymphadenopathy.
 (e) Presence of factor V Leiden.

21 Disseminated intravascular coagulation
 (a) Is commonly seen as a presenting feature of acute promyelocytic leukaemia.
 (b) Is usually associated with a raised platelet count.
 (c) Is usually associated with reduced fibrinogen levels.
 (d) Is usually associated with a prolonged APTT.
 (e) Is usually associated with a normal TT.

22 Features suggesting a population of haemopoietic cells are monoclonal include:
 (a) Reactive proliferation in response to infection.
 (b) Uniform presence of an oncogene mutation.
 (c) Demonstration of a common chromosomal abnormality.
 (d) Positive staining for CD13 antigen.
 (e) Presence of Howell Jolly bodies.

23 Thrombin
 (a) Is activated by heparin.
 (b) Promotes platelet aggregation.
 (c) Causes deficient platelet aggregation in von Willebrand's disease.
 (d) Is crosslinked by Factor XIII.
 (e) Is cleaved by plasmin.

24 Protein C
 (a) Levels are reduced in vitamin K deficiency.
 (b) Deficiency predisposes to skin necrosis after commencing oral anticoagulant therapy.
 (c) Levels are inversely related to protein S levels.
 (d) Levels are reduced in liver disease.
 (e) Deficiency is a risk factor for thrombosis.

25 Acute leukaemia in children
 (a) Is more likely to be lymphoid than myeloid.
 (b) Has a remission rate following chemotherapy of <50%.
 (c) Is more common in children with Down syndrome.
 (d) Carries a worse prognosis if presenting WBC is $>50 \times 10^9/L$.
 (e) May present with lytic bone lesions.

Answers
1 (a) False. MCV is usually low.
 (b) True.
 (c) False. Is most commonly due to bleeding.
 (d) True.
 (e) False. The rate of response is similar and related to time taken for haemopoiesis to occur (5–7 days).

2 (a) False. Renal failure is usually associated with a normochromic normocytic anaemia.
 (b) True, e.g. pernicious anaemia, vegetarianism, post gastrectomy.
 (c) False. The anaemia of chronic disease is normocytic or mildly microcytic.
 (d) True.
 (e) False.

3 (a) False.
 (b) False. Bone marrow failure = anaemia, leucopenia and thrombocytopenia. CML presents with leucocytosis, splenomegaly.
 (c) True. >95% of patients have the Philadelphia chromosome t(9;22).

(d) True.
(e) True.

4 (a) True.
(b) False.
(c) False. Median survival is 7–10 years.
(d) True. Up to 30% of patients.
(e) True. >95% are B cell.

5 (a) True.
(b) False.
(c) True.
(d) True.
(e) False. Monocytes often raised >1000 × 10⁹/L (chronic myelomonocytic leukaemia).

6 (a) False. Heparin is preferable during pregnancy. Warfarin is teratogenic.
(b) False. The INR is used to monitor Warfarin therapy.
(c) False.
(d) True. Protamine is used to reverse heparin.
(e) False. Three months, unless there are any other thrombosis risk factors.

7 (a) False. Factor VIII concentrate or recombinant factor VIII is used.
(b) False. It is not heat treated. Viral transmission can occur, although the risk is low.
(c) False. Corticosteroids, immunosuppressives, splenectomy and intravenous gammaglobulin.
(d) True, especially in conjunction with plasma exchange and if first depleted of cryoprecipitate.
(e) True.

8 (a) True. Due to transplacental passage of maternal IgG antibodies.
(b) True, e.g. congenital rubella, CMV.
(c) True, e.g. anti-HPA 1a antibodies.
(d) True. Due to half life of maternally derived antibodies.
(e) True. Thrombocytopenia with absent radii (TAR).

9 (a) False. Anaemia only occurs when marrow compensation fails.
(b) True.
(c) False. The anaemia is usually acholuric.
(d) True. Haemolysis occurs within the marrow and RES.
(e) True. This is due to deposition of unconjugated bilirubin in the neonatal brain.

10 (a) False. It is commonly seen in parasitic diseases.
(b) True.
(c) False. Basophilia is much more common.
(d) True.
(e) True.

11 (a) True.
(b) False. Thalassaemia trait occurs independently of pregnancy.
(c) True.
(d) True.

(e) False. Platelet count often lowered in pregnancy.

12 (a) False. Smokers can develop secondary or spurious polycythaemia.
(b) True. This is due to hyperuricaemia.
(c) True. Approximately 5% of cases.
(d) True. In 2/3 cases.
(e) True.

13 (a) False. They are a source of thromboxane.
(b) False. They do not have nuclei.
(c) True.
(d) True.
(e) True.

14 (a) False.
(b) True.
(c) True.
(d) False.
(e) True.

15 (a) False. It is sex-linked.
(b) False it is autosomal dominant.
(c) False. There is a 1:4 chance.
(d) True.
(e) True.

16 (a) True.
(b) False.
(c) False.
(d) True.
(e) False.

17 (a) False. Selected, poor risk patients only.
(b) False. Children generally tolerate the procedure better than adults.
(c) True.
(d) False. Blood products used in supportive care are irradiated.
(e) False. CMV infection is important, however.

18 (a) False. More commonly B cell.
(b) True.
(c) True.
(d) True.
(e) False. They are increasing.

19 (a) False.
(b) True.
(c) True.
(d) True.
(e) True.

20 (a) False. This is a red cell enzymopathy.
(b) True.
(c) True. As is chronic lymphocytic leukaemia.
(d) False.
(e) False. This is a risk factor for thrombosis.

21 (a) True.
   (b) False. The platelet count is usually low.
   (c) True.
   (d) True.
   (e) False. Usually prolonged.

22 (a) False. Reactive proliferations are usually polyclonal.
   (b) True.
   (c) True.
   (d) False.
   (e) False. These are found post splenectomy in red cells.

23 (a) False. Heparin activates antithrombin.
   (b) True.
   (c) False.
   (d) False.
   (e) False.

24 (a) True.
   (b) True.
   (c) False.
   (d) True.
   (e) True.

25 (a) True.
   (b) False. Remission rates for ALL and AML >90%.
   (c) True.
   (d) True.
   (e) True.

Case history 1

A 66-year-old caucasian man gives a history of increasing tiredness and lethargy over the preceding 2–4 months. He has recently lost his wife and has been drinking more alcohol than usual. His appetite is poor and he has lost 1 stone in weight over the past 3 months. He eats a mixed diet. His bowels are regular and he does not report any blood loss. He is not on any medication. He has not had any illnesses in the past.

On examination he is pale but not jaundiced. His blood pressure is 135/80. Abdominal examination, including rectal, is normal and there are no other abnormalities.

His FBC shows:
Hb = 7.6 g/dL
MCV = 68 fL
MCH = 26
WBC = 8.6 × 10^9/L
Platelets = 490 × 10^9/L
ESR = 83 mm/h

Questions
What is the differential diagnosis?
How would you manage him?

Answers
A history of anorexia and weight loss suggest occult malignancy. A microcytic anaemia suggests iron deficiency, and the elevated platelet count suggests bleeding as the cause. The raised ESR supports a diagnosis of underlying malignancy.

An accurate dietary and alcohol history should be taken, although alcohol usually causes a macrocytic anaemia. A poor diet may also cause folic acid or B$_{12}$ deficiency, which would also cause a macrocytic anaemia.

Management: diagnosis and treatment
Further diagnostic tests should include serum ferritin, serum B$_{12}$ and serum folate. Urea and electrolytes and liver function tests should also be done. A search for a cause of bleeding is mandatory, even though physical examination does not offer clues to the source of blood loss. Once iron deficiency is confirmed, endoscopic and/or radiological investigation of the GI tract is indicated.

The serum ferritin was reduced at 5 μg/L confirming iron deficiency. Upper GI endoscopy revealed a malignant gastric ulcer which was successfully resected.

Case history 2

A 71-year-old man has back pain. This has been present for over three months and is worse in the lower back. He has also developed upper abdominal pain and constipation over the last month. He has had no serious illnesses in the past. His appetite is poor and he has lost 1 stone in weight over the previous month. His medication includes pain killers (paracetamol and Ibuprofen).

On examination he is pale. His blood pressure is slightly elevated (160/100). Urine examinatin shows 2+ proteinuria.

Investigations show:

Hb = 8.6 g/dL
WBC = 9.5 × 10^9/L
Platelets = 65 × 10^9/L
ESR = 110 mm/h

Blood film report: Rouleaux
Leucoerythroblastic changes present

Questions
What is the differential diagnosis?
What further tests are indicated?

Answers
A history of recent onset of back pain, with poor appetite and weight loss, suggests malignant infiltration of the skeleton. Abdominal pain and constipation are suggestive of hypercalcaemia.

Proteinuria on urine testing suggests renal disease. There is no history of prostatic obstruction. The very high ESR suggests myeloma or carcinoma with bony metastases. Further tests should include urea and electrolytes, creatinine clearance, calcium level and serum alkaline phosphatase. X-rays of his back are required. Serum and urinary protein electrophoresis are needed to exclude myeloma.

A prostate specific antigen test to exclude prostatic carcinoma is required. This patient's calcium level was raised at 3.6 mmol/L and he was in renal failure (serum creatinine 860 mmol/L).

The serum alkaline phosphatase was normal, which is in keeping with multiple myeloma rather than secondary deposits. Skeletal survey, bone marrow, serum and urine paraprotein level, serum β_2 microglobulin are indicated (see Chapter 24).

Case history 3

A 64-year-old caucasian lady complains of gradually increasing tiredness. She feels the cold more than she used to. She also has a sore tongue. Over the past two months she has complained of numbness of her feet. Her sister suffers from hypothyroidism. She eats a normal diet.

On examination she is pale and very slightly jaundiced. Her tongue is reddened and enlarged; she has grey hair. The thyroid gland is clinically normal. She has reduced touch and joint position sense in the toes and the ankle jerks are absent. Neurological examination is otherwise normal.

Investigations show:

Hb = 6.4 g/dL
MCV = 131 fL

WBC = 3.1×10^9/L
Platelets = 63×10^9/L

Questions

What is the diagnosis?
Which further investigations are required?
How would you treat her?

Answer

This lady presents a classic clinical picture of pernicious anaemia (p. 37).

The further investigations required are listed on p. 38.

Treatment is with hydroxocobalamin (1 mg intramuscular) immediately followed by further B_{12} injections. It is important not to give folic acid before giving B_{12}, as it may precipitate neuropathy.

Index